Your Body Relationship

Overcoming Weight Obsession

Lemuela Christina Duskis M.Ed.

By Lemuela Christina Duskis M.Ed.
Copyright © 2014 by Lemuela Christina Duskis M.Ed.

The author of the book does not make any claim or guarantee for any physical, mental, emotional, or spiritual result. All products, services and information provided by the author are for general education and entertainment purposes only. The information provided herein is in no way a substitute for medical advice. In the event you use any of the information contained in this book for yourself, the author assumes no responsibility for your actions.

Editor: Christina Cutting
Cover author photo: A. Light Photography
Cover design: www.cosminviz.com / Cosmin Vizitiu
Front cover scale: www.shutterstock.com
Interior design: CreateSpace

ISBN: 1503017133
ISBN 13: 9781503017139
Library of Congress Control Number: 2014919403
CreateSpace Independent Publishing Platform
North Charleston, South Carolina

This book is dedicated to my father, Dr. Ronald Alan Duskis, who taught me the importance of giving kindness and love, and taught me all about having a relationship with God. I know he is with me every step of the way. His legacy lives on.

My vision is that men and women, adults and children, throughout the world, will know their worth and beauty because of who they are and who they be; an incredible, beautiful and lovable spirit; and that they love, nurture and honor their earthly home, their gift, their BODY.

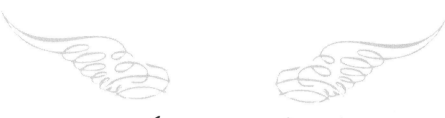

Gratitude

Thank you to my dear and special momma, Pina Tarlecki, who has been my greatest support in all things. I am grateful for her unconditional and constant love and care. I am filled with gratitude beyond words for who she is.

Thank you to my little sister, Charissa Joy Jones, who has been the greatest gift in my life! Thirty-two years ago, she became an answer to my prayers. Need I say anymore?

A special thank you to Dr. Lawrence Conlan for teaching me about being kind to myself and soaking into wherever I am in life. My heart overflows with gratitude.

Thank you to Dr. Anthony Page for all of the care he gave me when I lived in Italy. He forever holds a special place in my heart.

Thank you to Stephanie Hershey Schoolmeester for that pivotal moment when she told me to give myself grace, and for always being with me in a space of non-judgment. Non-judgment, it's a priceless gift! I bless the day we started teaching together.

Thank you to Erin Carroll Lausman for BEING and for all that I have learned from our countless talks over a glass of wine. Our friendship is a gift beyond measure!

Thank you to Candi Lee DeBlase for the years of laughter and support, and the knowing that no matter what, I've got a friend.

Thank you to Pina Tarlecki, Charissa Joy Jones, Erin Carroll Lausman, Stephanie Hershey Schoolmeester, and Julie Steinbeiss for being my book angels, for the constructive feedback, and for the continued support and unconditional love.

Thank you to Rachel Hartenstein and Julie Steinbeiss for listening to me talk about my book, a lot, and for their total support and friendship.

Thank you to my editor, Christina Cutting, for her beautiful and delicate work with my book.

Thank you to all of the special clients that I have had the privilege to serve. I am honored and I have learned so much from all of you.

Thank you to everyone who has supported me and encouraged me throughout this whole book writing process.

And gratitude to my sweet angels that are always with me, protecting me and helping me when I ask.

And finally, a special thank you to anyone who has crossed my path. Thank you for loving me in any way that you have. This whole life… it's all about the love!

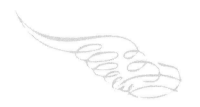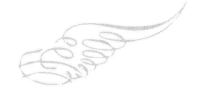

Just as You Are

There is nothing wrong with you.
There never was anything wrong with you.
There never will be anything wrong with you.

You are a beautiful being just as you are.
You are a magical, powerful and intuitive being.
You are perfect just as you are.

You are lovable.
You are loved.
You are pure love.

You are a gift.
You are a gift in other people's lives.
You are a gift in your life.

There is nothing wrong with you.
There never was anything wrong with you.
There never will be anything wrong with you.
You are perfect just as you.

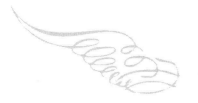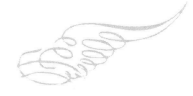

Contents

Disclaimer

The information in this book is solely my opinion based on my experience. Any time you make a change to your diet, your lifestyle, or your thinking, you should consult with a medical doctor first. I am not a doctor and everything that I have written in this book is purely my opinion and point of view based on my experiences.

I invite you to join the free virtual book club for
Your Body Relationship: Overcoming Weight Obsession.

Sign up at www.lemuelachristina.com

I look forward to personally connecting with you through
Facebook, tele-calls, videos, articles, and more on how
you can continue to build a healthy and happy
relationship with your body.

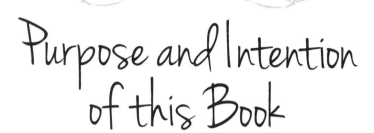

Purpose and Intention of this Book

My purpose in writing this book is to share with others who face the day to day challenge of constantly worrying about their weight, tools that I have acquired through my journey in a battle against my weight.

What started out as an innocent diet at the age of 11, led to a life-long battle of chronic yo-yo dieting, starving, binging and purging, and lots and lots of self-loathing. I have participated in a 12-step program, I have been an out-patient at a clinic, I have gone through psychotherapy, hypnotherapy, read books and any other thing I could get my hands on to alleviate the mental insanity that plagued my every thought about my body.

Along the way, I began to take pieces from all of the programs and books and found what worked for me. Here in this book I will share with you my experiences and all of the tools, ideas, and strategies that have collectively worked for me. At the age of 36 years old, I can say I love my body, appreciate my body, and have a beautiful relationship with my body. I am confident I will never be in a battle with my weight and my body again, as long as I continue to use the tools outlined in this book.

My intention is that you too will find tools that you can use to love your body and yourself. Most importantly, my hope is that you learn how to build a relationship with your body, because when you do, your whole world gets better in every aspect, including your relationships with others, your career, and how you respond to the outside world.

My hope for you is that you thrive in life, that you love in life, and that you can get through life's storms and joys with calm; knowing that you are always taken care of.

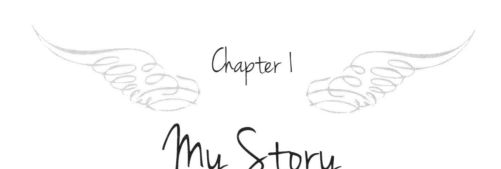

Chapter 1

My Story

I was 11 years old when I went on my first diet. I remember clearly going to the weight loss center to get weighed in and attend meetings. You're probably wondering how overweight I was at such a young age to have been part of a weight loss program. At my first weigh in, I was 112 pounds.

I was 11 years old.

I was 5 foot tall.

I weighed 112 pounds.

They let me go on a diet. They, meaning every responsible adult, who really were only doing what they thought was right based on what they had learned from other adults in our society and the media.

I've seen the pictures of myself at this time in my life. I wasn't fat. I wasn't anywhere near fat. I wasn't even chunky or soft. I was just an 11-year-old girl that had picked up the idea from somewhere that there was something wrong with her, an 11-year-old girl who had certain concerns and beliefs that she had picked up from the adults around her and the media.

My journey with food, body image, and weight began here.

My target weight that they set for me was 103 pounds. I can still see myself waiting in line behind the others, like a big cattle call, and then finally getting on the professional medical scale, the big silver kind where you wait for the balance bar to even out and tell you what your number is, and having that anticipation of, *Did I do it or not?*

I also remember being hungry.

I lost about 5 pounds from this program.

I also gained those 5 pounds back.

Not too long after this, I went on another diet. I had a shake for breakfast, a shake for lunch, and then I ate a small dinner. I chose this diet because I saw a commercial for it practically every time I watched TV. I also wanted to lose 5 pounds, and I wanted to lose those 5 pounds quickly. Well, I did!

I remember being hungry, very hungry.

I didn't go on my next official diet until I was 14 years old. In between those couple of years, I had just kind of given up and decided that I was a chunky girl, and that was the way it was. At some point though, I reached a place where I was so frustrated with my weight, because I wasn't as thin as I wanted to be, that I felt hopeless. I felt embarrassed about my weight. I just wanted to be thin.

I decided one day that I was not going to eat anything except for a couple of crackers a day. That lasted a few hours, and then I ate the whole box of crackers! I remember feeling very surprised at myself for eating so quickly and so much.

Not too long after, I was introduced to an herbal weight loss supplement from a very well-known multi-level marketing company. It worked! I rapidly dropped about 15 pounds. My appetite was almost nil. I was hardly eating. I was a very happy 14-year-old girl.

For the next few years, I often relied on weight loss supplements, but nothing seemed to work quite like the first time. I had success with it that first time. But, even when I had gone back and tried that same product, it just didn't have the same effect on my appetite like it had before. I wasn't dropping the weight as quickly. I just wasn't seeing results like I did the first time. I wondered what was wrong with me. I increased my dosage, so as to decrease my appetite, and I began to experience heart palpitations and short bouts of blacking out. That scared me enough that I swore off all diet pills that had a thermogenic effect. What that means is I turned to alternative pills. Pills that promised to block a certain percentage of carbohydrates, and pills that supposedly would block the fat from food. I became frustrated with those, because they didn't seem to work for me either.

My weight continued to fluctuate throughout my teenage years, until I hit college, where I discovered working out consistently and counting my calories. I exercised every day and ate between 500-800 calories a day. I thought that I had finally mastered it. I even measured out my peas, carrots, and corn. I weighed in at 97 pounds, and I was a very, very hungry girl.

I was passing judgment all the time on everyone else for eating and for not being as thin as me. Can you believe I was judging people for eating? I was always comparing myself to the girls who I thought were skinnier than me, and wondering how they got there, and comparing myself to the girls who were bigger, thinking how afraid I was of ever gaining any weight back.

In college, my weight fluctuated anyway. I know these numbers precisely because I was so crazed at the time about them. When I was no longer satisfied with being 97-103 pounds and thought I could lose just a little more, I tried the no carb diet, which worked great while I was on it, but the moment I even thought about sinking my teeth into a carb such as a piece of bread, I was toast. I was off and running like I hadn't eaten in years! But, I guess, I hadn't truly eaten in years.

I began to understand what the term yo-yo dieting meant. I understood that I was a yo-yo dieter, but I had no intention of living any other way. I used to joke, "All I ever wanted in life was to be thin," but we all know that there is always some truth in a joke.

I knew I meant it. I really couldn't imagine being happy unless I was thin, but I was never thin enough, so I was always focused on my weight. In short, I was never happy with my weight and my body.

When standing in line at the grocery store, I would buy 2-3 magazines at a time, ones that promised weight loss if I followed their weekly menus or did their weekly workout routines. I bought the pills that were advertised in those magazines. The ones that promised they had found the breakthrough cure to melt fat once and for all from some special flower that was miraculously discovered in the Amazon!

I spent thousands of dollars on my quest to be a thinner me. It never mattered how thin I was or not, because I never thought I was thin enough. I was never satisfied with my body, but this was something I wouldn't realize until many years later.

During my senior year in college, my boyfriend and I broke up after five years of dating. I went out every night with friends and lived up my new found freedom. I drank a lot. I ate almost every night at two in the morning, when I would come home from the bars. I put on weight rapidly, and I began to really hate myself. Every day I would say that I wasn't going to do that again and every night I would.

Shortly after I graduated from Colorado State University with a degree in Psychology, I moved to San Diego, California. Alone and on my own for the first time at the age of 23, I found that I had lost complete control of my ability to control my weight. I couldn't stop eating. I just couldn't stop eating. I would stand at the fridge telling myself, "Just one more bite."

I couldn't stop eating until I could no longer eat because my stomach was in so much pain. I was terrified of the weight I had put on. I was then tipping the scales at 138 pounds. Within a matter of months, I had put on nearly 40 pounds. I was devastated; I was ashamed, and I was embarrassed. I was out of control, and I knew it.

I knew something had to be done, so I turned to laxatives and throwing up the food that I had overindulged in. I felt like something was wrong with me. I knew that I had gone overboard, but I didn't know how to stop; all that mattered to me was losing the weight I had gained. I felt hopeless.

One afternoon when I had arrived back to my apartment in San Diego, I checked the mail, and as I was going through it, I came across a flier that was geared towards people who compulsively overeat. I knew that I was one of those people. I knew that anyone who sticks their fingers down their throat has a serious issue. I knew that something wasn't right. I knew I couldn't continue to live like this anymore and that I didn't want to live like this any longer. I knew that I needed help, and so I responded to the flier.

This was the beginning of my journey of healing my relationship with food. Although I learned a few valuable tools from this program, it still wasn't enough for me. I still felt out of control with food. I still felt fat. I still felt frustrated. However, this program introduced me to the possibility of being helped and the possibility of recovering from an all-consuming obsession with weight and body image.

I began searching for more answers. I began reading books on compulsive overeating. I went to talk therapy, hypnotherapy, and I joined a 12-step program.

But still there was something in me that was still not satisfied with my weight and still not satisfied with my body. I yearned so much to be skinny like I once was. I just felt that if I could lose the weight, then I could return to a normal lifestyle and eat and think like normal people do.

There is a very popular newspaper in San Diego that comes out once a week, and I would read all of the ads that promised a perfectly sculpted body. They all suggested that liposuction was the way to go. For a while, I contemplated if this was something I should do or not. One day, I decided that the only way for me to lose weight was to have liposuction. I was 23 years old.

I was 23 years old. Isn't that crazy?

I was 138 pounds.

I was 5 foot and 1 inch.

You know what's crazier?

You know what's sadder?

You know what's even scarier?

It's that the doctor didn't turn me away.

He didn't say that I was too young. He didn't say that I should see a therapist or a nutritionist or seek counseling. He accepted me as his next liposuction patient.

I was 23 years old when I opened up a line of credit on a credit card with a 0% percent interest rate for a year and charged $5,000 so that I could have fat sucked out from my thighs, my ass, my arms, my stomach, and under my chin. I went from a size 9 to a size 3 within about a week after the swelling went down.

What I found in the days, weeks and months after, was that I still needed my 12-step program. My desire to eat wasn't sucked away with the fat cells from the liposuction. I was still me. I still had the same thoughts and compulsions. I continued to work the 12-step program and attend meetings, but I never told anyone that I had surgery to lose weight. I was embarrassed about the fact that I had stooped to that level.

Going under the knife to lose weight is not one of my prouder moments, but nevertheless, it is something that has already been done.

Would I take it back? No. I believe every experience is part of our journey. I have since apologized to my beautiful body for voluntarily putting it through something so invasive and unkind.

It took courage for me to write about the liposuction here. Before writing this book and teaching the classes I teach on how to love your body, there were a handful of people who knew about the liposuction I had.

I believe that if I am going to effect change, I must be brutally honest. We all must be. We all need to stop hiding the truth and start talking about it.

Do you think I kept the weight off after I had the liposuction? Do you think I finally got *there*? After spending $5,000 and going through surgery for it, one would think so, right? Well, I didn't. My weight stayed fairly steady for a few years because I was working the 12-step program, purging only on occasion, and I got into a routine of eating only certain foods at certain times, and I had stopped weighing myself.

One day, a few years later, I started weighing myself again, which led me to start binging again and I went back up to a size 9. Talk about devastation! I hired a personal trainer, worked out two hours a day, and stuck to a 1300 calorie a day diet to lose the weight…again!

After re-losing the post-lipo weight, I stopped purging, making a commitment to myself that if I was going to eat something, I was going to keep it down. I began following a set of tools that I had compiled over the years and finally became serious about using them. I would say the obsession had worn off, but still, what I ate and how I looked mattered immensely to me.

Then, something miraculously shifted within me at the age of 31. I had enough of all of it! I was tired. I was exhausted from 20 years of starving, dieting, binging, purging, and every thought and consideration that I had revolving around my weight. I'd had enough! I wanted out! I didn't want to hate myself anymore. I didn't want to be chained down by the thoughts and patterns that had ruled me for more than half of my life.

I noticed that there were times in my life when I wasn't dieting, that I hadn't gained any weight. I began eating for my health. I began loving my body as it was. I came up with a set of questions before I ate, and I looked at my beliefs and values around food. I crafted something that worked for me based on everything I had learned along the way in my journey. I became very presently aware of the way I was thinking about food, my body, and my weight. I began communicating with my body and listening to it.

I made a decision to give it a real shot to let go of everything that I had been doing for the past 20 years and to try something new. It was like a huge weight had been lifted off of me, and I was truly living life in a brand new way. It wasn't long before I realized that I wasn't thinking about food, my body, or my weight anymore. It wasn't an issue. Every day I thanked God for the freedom.

I stopped fighting my body. My clothes became loose on me, and people started asking me what I had done to lose weight. The only thing I had really done was stop trying to lose weight and control my body. I had given up. I had surrendered.

In June of 2013, I moved to Rome, Italy, for six months to study at an Italian language school. The idea for this book came to me as I was pondering what to do with my free time in Italy. My classes were in the morning and ended at 12:40. I didn't want to get a job, since one of my purposes for the time off of work was to simply enjoy the leisure time, but I didn't want to have too much free time on my hands either. As I wondered what to do with my afternoons, the idea came to me to share my story.

When I decided to write this book, I asked myself, *How did I over-come my weight obsession? How did I get to this place where I love my body? Really? How did that happen?*

After much reflection on those questions, I realized that it was due to all of the tools that I had learned along the way in my journey, the tools that I had created that worked for me, but one other observation stood out to me, this was all due to my relationship with my body. I realized that the key factor that allowed me to be free from my weight obsession was the relationship that I built with my body.

My gift now is to share with you all of the tools that I have learned and how to build a relationship with your body. You CAN have freedom from worrying about your weight. It is possible. The tools I share in this book work incredibly well to help with breaking the cycle of abuse and creating freedom from weight obsession.

If I could do it: starver, binger, purger, liposuction girl – then you can do it too. I know it! I believe in you, even if you don't! I believe that if you practice the tools in this book, it is inevitable that you will see shifts occur in the way you think about your body and food. Awareness creates change.

It wasn't until I had received some energy body work from a special chiropractor in Boulder, Colorado, that I learned to connect with my body and communicate with it. It was during this experience that I discovered the relationship that I have with my body. This understanding changed everything!

It was never the food or my weight that was the issue. There was nothing wrong with me or my body. It was what I **believed** about food, about my weight, and about my body that was the issue. People who eat normally don't share the same beliefs as people who obsess over their weight. Listen to the way people talk about food. Listen to their points of views and to what they believe, and realize that's all they are, points of views and beliefs that they have made true in their own world and reality.

My healing journey with food and my body continues; I believe it is a lifelong journey because I have a relationship with both. Relationships are never perfect; they go through ups and downs, and sometimes they change. However, I have learned how to communicate and appreciate my relationship with my body and food, and this has made all the difference. What I do know is that I am very aware now if any old beliefs or old thought patterns begin to show up. I recognize them instantly, and I know what to do. I also know that I don't have to worry about freedom from an obsession about food and weight for the rest of my life; I only need to be present within today.

In the following pages, I share with you all of the tools and strategies that I have learned and used in order to break free from the unhappy lifestyle that revolved around my weight.

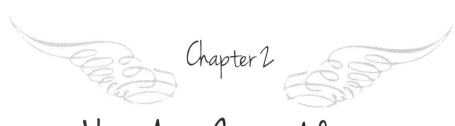

Chapter 2

You Are Not Alone

When I have conversations with people, I am amazed by the astonishing number of people who fight their weight on a daily basis. I was trying to count how many people I know that battle their weight in one way, or another. When I use the term battle, I mean that they are consciously trying to lose weight or stay thin. Then I started thinking of all of the celebrities, and also of all the people that I don't know, and I wondered, is it almost everyone? Are most people unhappy with their weight, their shape, or their body, whether it's 2 pounds, 10 pounds, 50 pounds?

Weight battles have become an epidemic in America. According to *Prevalence of Obesity in the United States, 2009-2010* study by the Centers for Disease Control and Prevention, 36% of people under the age of 20 are overweight or obese and 69% over the age of 20 are overweight or obese in America. (Cynthia L. Ogden, Margaret D. Carroll and Brian K. Kit 2012)

There are more books, diets, and diet supplements than ever before. In 2012, according to a wide range of statistics found across the internet, the public spent an estimated 40-65 billion dollars on weight loss, including gyms, diet sodas, diet products, weight loss programs, and bypass surgeries, just to name a few.

I, myself, am guilty of contributing to these statistics, as I have spent thousands and thousands of dollars in years past on a miracle, a quick fix, or a promise to lose weight if I followed a particular program.

Often, with certain groups of girls that I know, the conversation always circles its way back around to weight. While this may be a very "normal" or accepted conversation in the female population, it is most certainly not normal in my opinion. In fact, when I began to love my body and trust my body, I began to find these conversations extremely boring. Why? Because food and the obsession with being skinny no longer exists for me. I have lost interest in the subject.

It's important to know that you are not alone. It's important for people to talk about how they can help themselves and each other love their bodies, not how they can abuse their bodies by taking on another fad diet that will put them in a state of deprivation, throwing themselves back into the weight loss/weight gain cycle.

People need support from each other, and when they receive that support, they often flourish and overcome their addictions. This is why 12-step support programs work so well for so many people.

One of the problems in our society is that we don't talk about things. Our society is so afraid of the truth or of "hurting" other people's feelings that we stay mum about everything. When we don't talk, we stay in secret and in shame. When people talk and share their vulnerabilities, change happens. There is strength, power, and change in being vulnerable. There is loneliness in appearing strong.

People are afraid to share. Everyone wants to look good and to appear as if they've got their shit together. People want to be envied, so they buy a car that costs too much, or live in a house that is outside of their means, or beat themselves up and restrict themselves to unhealthy dieting so that others can look at them in awe of how amazing they are. People want other people to validate them and to validate their worthiness.

What matters is how amazing you think you are. What matters is the relationship that you have with your body. Is it kind? Is it loving? Would you treat the person you love most in this world, the way you treat yourself? Would you talk to them the way you talk to yourself?

I began loving my body a year after I started my mantra, "My body is beautiful, I love my body."

I found myself talking about how I was being kind to my body and not what weight I had gained or lost. I began changing the things I talked about and the conversations that I contributed to.

Knowing that so many in this world struggle with their weight, and with loving their body, is it possible to begin changing your conversations around it when it comes up?

What contribution to change can you be?

When your friends start talking about the next diet that they are going to try, can you start talking about what you are doing to honor your body? Lead by example, but no more talking about how to lose weight and how to deprive or hurt your body!

When I did this, my friends and family listened to me. They asked me more about the changes I was making. They too wanted help from the insanity of hating their bodies. Sharing my experience and changes with them brought them a new awareness and helped them heal their relationship with their bodies. My mom has told me numerous times that before she was going to eat something, she could hear me in her head, saying: *What can I choose that will make me feel good about what I have eaten after I have eaten it?*

We must be the change together; because, as a society, we have bought into the points of view that we are not good enough unless we look a certain way or weigh a certain amount. We must start selling a new idea that our bodies are a precious gift that our spirit calls home on earth, and that our body deserves to be treated with love, kindness, and gratitude.

Chapter 3

Tools

The way I have turned my weight obsession around is not a quick fix. It is a lifestyle that creates and leads to freedom from weight obsession! It is a lifestyle that results in weight loss naturally, and that leads to a healthy weight based on where your body wants to be. It is with a set of tools that I have compiled and created that I use every day. EVERY day I still use these tools. They have replaced my old and unhealthy habits and ways of thinking.

Here is a list of some of the tools I practice:

- I speak kindly to myself.
- I ask my body what it would like to eat before every meal.
- I am aware of the foods that feel good in my body and the foods which don't.
- I don't buy foods that were once triggers for me to overeat.
- I don't exercise to lose weight. I exercise because it makes me feel good to move, to take care of my heart, and to keep my muscles strong so that when I am older I can still move about and enjoy life.
- I pray over my food every time I eat because I believe in the mind-body connection and a higher power than myself.
- I thank my food for the gift that it is.

- I buy clothes that fit me now when I go shopping, because this is the size my body is today, and I wouldn't wear something that makes me feel yucky.
- If I eat something that does not make me feel good about my choice, I forgive myself and remind myself of the importance of being aware of what I choose.
- I sit down to eat my meals whenever possible and appreciate the nourishment that is before me.
- I am educated on foods and how they serve my body.
- My lifestyle choices are based on my beliefs and not on how they will affect my weight.
- I do not weigh or measure myself, and I am happy never to know those numbers again.
- I don't count calories.
- I choose not to read magazines with weight loss gimmicks, ads, and the promotion of super skinny people.
- I appreciate what my body does for me.
- When I eat, I eat for the present meal and that meal only.
- I have a relationship with my body.

This is my lifestyle. This is what I do every day.

Did it take conscious effort in the beginning? You bet your ass it did. It wasn't always easy, but it has become second nature now because I continue to practice and use the tools that work for me. I will say this though; there have been times in my life when I have felt myself slipping back to old thought patterns. For example, when I quit smoking cigarettes, I began to have thoughts about my weight again. I had to remind myself that quitting smoking doesn't put on weight; it's how we treat our body that puts on the weight. Smoking is a whole other addiction, in and of itself, and I had to relearn and shift many things in my thinking and lifestyle patterns when I first quit smoking.

When I notice my mind going back to old patterns, I STOP and slow down and take extra care to use the tools I have acquired along the way, and I always, always forgive myself.

I have a saying I came up with, "Forgive yourself for what you would do anyway."

I found forgiving myself for my choices took the power away from continuing the abusive cycle, because I could not and cannot change the past. I can only move forward.

You know yourself better than anyone out there. You know your body better than anyone else, but you have to listen to it and build that relationship with your body. At one time, my relationship with my body was that of a stranger or of a very, very broken relationship. I know how to build a strong body relationship, and I will teach you how through the tools in this book.

Is every day perfect for me? Of course not, and that's okay. I'll give you an example. I was on vacation in St. Barth's the summer my sister got married and St. Barth's is very expensive! It is probably one of the most expensive places I have ever traveled to. I didn't want to pay the high prices for the food because I felt that I couldn't afford it or didn't want to afford it.

The first day there I had a croissant for breakfast, pizza for lunch, and then pizza again for dinner because those were the cheapest options. By the end of the day I felt lethargic and bloated, and then I remembered, I didn't ask my body what it wanted. I made a choice based on price and not the needs of my body. I told myself, *Okay, remember this and choose your next meal based on what your body wants and not your pocketbook.*

The next morning, my mom and I found a café that had fresh salads and I paid the 10 euros for a small side salad and that's what I had for breakfast because my body wanted it. When we were at one of the trendy beach resorts, I ordered the 20 euro basic sushi roll, because that's what my body wanted. When we went to dinner, I listened to what my body was asking for and I ordered the 35 euro cod.

I didn't freak out that a day full of breads would make me gain weight. I just became aware that the choice I had made did not make me feel physically good, and I moved on.

As I sit here, I am beginning to get very hungry. This morning for breakfast I had a salad with rice and olive oil, for lunch I had a piece of pizza from my favorite little pizza shop down the street, and now I am going to step out and head to the grocery store because my body wants another salad and some salmon. I don't feel like leaving my apartment right now, but the current selection of food in my place is pasta, potatoes, eggs, and pizza, and this is not what my body wants. If I were to make a choice from what I have at home right now, I probably wouldn't feel good about it. I will honor my body and take myself to the store to pick up the nourishment it requires of me and asks of me.

I eat what I want, when I want it. For most of my life, I held the belief that certain foods were bad for me, that they would make me gain weight. I eat more pizza and French fries now, than I did when I was dieting, and I am happier with my body than I have ever been.

It's very interesting how, for years, I spent so much time and energy dieting, starving, binging, purging, hating myself and always preoccupied with thoughts about my weight and the only difference in my body now from those years when I tried to control it, is that my weight has stabilized to a normal, healthy weight and I am free of the insanity. If only I had known, it was me that was holding me back.

Chapter 4

Diets Don't Work

Diets don't work! Google it! At least they don't have a lasting effect. The problem with dieting is that it is a temporary action with a temporary result. Most people go on a diet to fix something that is wrong with them. Well, I am here to tell you that there is nothing wrong with you! The only reason you would think that you need to be fixed is because the media and our society have marketed a bunch of belief systems and you bought into them!

The belief system being fed to you over and over by the media and through your interactions with others is that you are not good enough unless you look a certain way. When you buy into these lies, you feel bad about your body.

You may think;

I'm too fat.

I'm too thin.

My knees are sagging.

I have a muffin top.

If I could just get rid of this back fat...

I have too many lines around my eyes.

My eyelashes aren't long enough.

Etc...

We can beat up and pick on any part of our body we choose, but we got the idea to do so from somewhere else.

For example, you see a magazine that advertises on its front cover:
Get Rid of Jiggly Arms

You go home, hold up an arm in the mirror and wave, and then think, *I've got jiggly arms, and I need to get rid of that.*

You have just been sold a belief.

We acquire many beliefs about our body in this way, and that's just one measly example.

Most people start out on the dieting path innocently. They don't intend to make it a life-long career, but what happens is this:

They are unhappy with some part of their body or their weight and so they go on a diet and restrict their food intake. They begin following guidelines on how they should eat.

Then one of two things happen, or both:

1) They lose weight and go back to their old ways of eating and doing things. Perhaps they indulge a little since they were deprived on their diet and think that since they have lost the weight they wanted to, that they can indulge just this one time.

2) They fall off the wagon while they are on the diet and for all of the food they deprived themselves of, they now eat, and more. They then go back to their old patterns of eating.

In both scenarios, they regain the lost weight, usually adding a few more pounds on their body than before they went on the diet in the first place. Feeling really bad about being back to where they were and putting on additional weight, they beat themselves up emotionally for it. They feel like a failure, they feel not good enough, not hot enough, not beautiful enough, and not lovable. Finding themselves feeling unhappy with their body and their weight again, they find another diet, a program, or a diet pill to help them lose the weight. They vow that this time they will stick to it for good, and vow that they will never ever eat bad foods again. They have a fierce sense of determination and the best of intentions. So they follow their program, take their pills, exercise in the morning and again at night, pass up on the foods they enjoy and eat what they are told they should eat.

There is a moment that comes when they are at a birthday party and everyone's having cake or they're at a BBQ and everyone's eating cheeseburgers, that they say, "Just this once I'll have a piece of cake," or, "Just this once, I'll have a cheeseburger," and so they do.

Then they feel guilty; that icky, yucky sensation that they are a bad person and have done something absolutely horrible, and now their entire diet is ruined.

So, they do one of two things:

1) They punish themselves. They cut back even more on their food intake the following day and they throw in an extra hour of cardio on top of the one and a half hours they are already doing.

2) They say, "Fuck it, I've already messed up and blown it," and continue to eat everything they think is bad, until they are numb from true emotion because they can only feel how full their stomach is. They go back to their old patterns of eating, regain any lost weight, plus more, give themselves an emotional beating for failing again and still being fat and imperfect, until the day rolls around again when they believe a promise from another program, diet, or pill, that says they can be the perfect them if they follow the program. The cycle continues, and with each new diet, more weight is put on. It becomes a battle, a fight. This is what I call *The Abuse Your Body Cycle* (page 20).

Diets don't work in the long term for weight loss and happiness, and there are tons of statistics and studies to support that.

What does work? You have most likely heard that a healthy lifestyle works, but how do you know that when you have been taught a million different ways on what to eat, what not to eat, what is healthy, what isn't healthy, what is good, and what is bad?

Well, it starts with the *Love Your Body Cycle*. *The Love Your Body Cycle* is the opposite of what the media teaches you and what you hear people saying. *The Love Your Body Cycle* doesn't start with what you should and shouldn't do. It starts with you, and you connecting to your body and spirit, communicating, honoring, and being kind.

It works like this:

You treat your body with kindness; you give it kind messages, being aware of your old thought patterns, while working to change them. You honor your body by taking care of it, asking it what it needs from you today and then listening to how your body responds. This builds trust in your relationship with your body that is probably not there right now. When you begin to trust your body and your body begins to trust that you will take care of it and be kind to it, your relationship with your body grows. This, in turn, makes you love your body and respect it. When you love your body and respect it, you naturally want to do good things for it, you naturally want to treat your body with kindness, and ask it what it wants and listen to it.

The Love Your Body Cycle (page 21) is simple, and the way to get into that cycle is pretty simple too, and that's what this book is about. It's about learning how to be kind to your body, honor your body, and communicate with it, which is what I call the three simple steps to building a healthy and happy relationship with your body.

The Abuse Your Body Cycle

You are unhappy with your body and your weight

You go on a diet or restrict your food intake

You lose weight/Fall off the wagon

You go back to old patterns of eating

You regain the lost weight

You beat yourself up emotionally for failing

The Love Your Body Cycle

You love your body

You are kind to your body

You honor your body

You communicate with your body

You trust your body

Your relationship with your body grows

Chapter 5

Acknowledging Your Thoughts

If you are obsessed with your weight, it is more likely than not that you have an endless amount of chatter happening in your brain related to food and weight. This can also be looked at as a form of anxiety, something that does not give you peace, but quite the opposite, it keeps you in a state of being that is quite uncomfortable.

If you use the tools I have laid out in this book, you will find that a lot of that obsession and chatter tends to fall away naturally. Finding your present can also help with this. Often when people's minds are racing, they are not thinking about what they are doing now or where they are now, they are thinking either about the past or about the future, but they are not in their present. Their minds are floating away so to speak. In order for people to avoid their present, they let their mind wander away with the chatter.

You may say, "Let? I don't let my mind chatter with thoughts. I can't control what it thinks," but, at one time, my dear friend, you did not chatter in your head nonstop about such things as your weight. Over time, you have allowed your thoughts to continue to repeat themselves, and now it feels that you have lost control, but you haven't. You just have to retrain your brain.

Sometimes, finding one's present can be challenging, but I have found that the simplest way to be present is to go towards whatever it is that I am feeling. What I mean by that is, instead of trying to change what I am thinking about, I say to myself, *Okay, right now I keep thinking about... and that's okay.* It's about being in allowance instead of resisting.

All of my very close friends know that I have a tendency to say very often, and about many different feelings and situations, "...and that's okay."

You know why? Because it is, it really usually is.

I am sure you have heard of the saying, "What you resist, persists."

This is so very true. If you resist the thoughts that you have, they will continue to come at you, but if you go towards them with love, they will have no choice but to melt into your kindness and grace.

Try acknowledging your thoughts and feelings. You can tell yourself something like, *I am aware that it feels like my brain is on a runaway train; thinking about how I look, or how much I ate, or how I will lose the next five pounds.*

Now, sit there and observe what you notice. Did your body take a big breath? Did you let out a sigh? Did your body relax? Did your mind feel understood? Chances are when you acknowledged how you felt about your thoughts, it brought some kind of relief to your body and your mind, because instead of being unkind to that part of you and fighting it, you were aware of it, you embraced it, and you accepted it for what it was, for just being there. These racing thoughts are a part of you trying to get your attention, by saying, *Hey, there is something you need to acknowledge right now that you are not acknowledging.*

Awareness creates change; it is inevitable.

After this acknowledgment, you can ask, *Body what are you trying to tell me?*

You don't have to figure anything out, just asking and communicating in a relationship with your body is enough. It's similar to when you are in a relationship and your significant other keeps nagging at you that you are not spending enough time together. Their nagging is really annoying and you wish they would just stop pestering you, but one day you stop and listen because you are so tired of their endless chatter about you not spending time with them and you say kindly, "I hear you, you would like to spend more time together. Let me know how we can make that happen," and as soon as you stop, listen and respond, they relax and stop nagging you.

If you make time for your relationship with your body, it will stop nagging you, it will stop yelling at you.

Almost everything I talk about doing to free yourself from body and weight obsession is the opposite of what we do when we are in the obsession, and this makes sense if you think about it. People who give up smoking, stop smoking, and live in a new way that does not involve smoking. People who choose not to drink anymore, stop drinking, and live in a new way that does not involve drinking; people who stop obsessing about their weight, stop dieting, and stop revolving their life around food. It may not be easy, but it can be done, and when you get over the initial stage of letting your old habits go, and you begin to trust your body, it all flows with more ease.

You cannot hold onto the idea of controlling your weight, without the consequences of your brain thinking about food, your weight, and diets all of the time, just as a smoker cannot smoke without the consequences of a cough or some other physical symptom. This is why I highly suggest using tools such as avoiding certain magazines and the scale.

I am sure many people who have given up cigarettes or alcohol or gambling or whatever it is they have felt a loss of power over, have at times had to acknowledge, "I would really like a drink/a cigarette/to play a poker game... right now, I really would, but I am choosing not to."

Acknowledgement is powerful and simple. The reason dieting becomes so hard is because people are trying to control what is happening with their bodies instead of listening, being aware of, and acknowledging what is happening. Dieting and trying to control what happens with our bodies creates a separation between spirit and body which is only brought back together with the ease of communicating and being present.

There is no mind control that is going to change the shape of your body so that you become thinner, but acknowledging what is happening in your mind, with your spirit, and in your body, will create harmony within you and this harmony creates ease in your body and mind, and thus, results in a body that is happy, at peace, at ease, and is pleasing to your eyes.

Next time you are aware that your mind is wandering obsessively about your weight, or about what you will eat or cannot eat, say out loud or in your head, "Body and mind what do you need from me right now? What are you trying to tell me? I hear that you are trying to let me know something."

Then, let it go. If you hear something or feel something, awesome; if you don't, that is okay too. What is important, and what helps, is that you acknowledge your present thoughts.

Chapter 6

Value

What value are you putting on your weight? The value you are putting on your weight has become a part of your belief system. Just because something is a part of your belief system, does not make it an absolute fact. This makes it a point of view that you have created and accepted as true for you.

Does your weight make you a different person? An unworthy person? An unlovable person? Does it change who you are inside? Does it change your heart? Does it change that you love? Does it change the things you like? The answer is no. Your weight does not change who you are. Your point of view on your weight affects the way you respond to life. The way you respond to life affects the way others respond to you. Your weight is not the issue; your perception is.

In one *The Love Your Body Class* that I taught, someone said they believed that people who are overweight are scary. The other classmates were a little taken aback by this point of view. I too had never thought of someone as scary just because of their weight. This belief was feeding a value my student had about her weight. As we discussed this point of view, my student discovered it was her way of protecting herself so that she would not have to be too close to people. If she were scary, people would need to keep their distance from her, or vice versa.

During a one-on-one *The Love Your Body Retreat*, another one of my clients discovered that she put on weight to protect herself from a man that she was with, from him wanting her, and she kept the weight on to protect herself from ever attracting another man like that, one who was not always kind to her.

And during another one-on-one *The Love Your Body Retreat,* my client discovered that she was carrying around extra weight because she was holding on to a family issue that went back to her father cheating on her family. She didn't want to be too attractive and cheat on her husband and then lose the family that she had created. This was the value she had put on being overweight, but she had no idea that she was carrying around a certain set of beliefs until I had asked her some questions to unlock them.

So, what is it that you are getting out of your frustration with your weight? What are you getting out of counting calories and trying new fad diets? What is the value? What's underneath there? I always say it's not about the weight. We don't feel fat. We feel not good enough. We feel insecure. We feel worried. We feel sad. We mask these feelings by feeling fat.

For me, it was a few things. It was a way of living that I knew, and it was a way of living that was familiar. It was also something that bonded me to my mother and my friends. It reinforced my belief that I was not good enough. In the rare instance that I feel fat comes up again, I always ask myself:

What's underneath that?

What am I really feeling?

What value and purpose is this serving right now?

See if you can answer the following question on a piece of paper.

What value are you getting out of worrying about your weight and trying to control it?

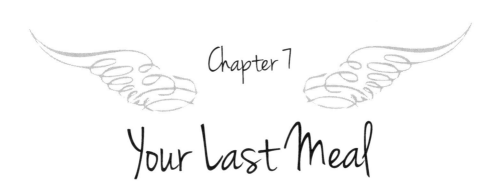

Chapter 7

Your Last Meal

Have you ever felt like the meal you are eating is your last meal? If so, you were probably getting ready to go on a diet, or you had "blown" your diet. You figured you might as well eat whatever you want at this meal, or today, or on vacation, or whatever time span you agreed with yourself that it was okay to eat everything and anything.

Sometimes a last meal is like, "I am going to eat a pizza, the chips, and the cookies, and then I will not eat anything with carbs anymore. That's it; I'm done."

It is a form of bargaining with yourself so that you feel justified to eat the food that you feel completely deprived of.

I, myself, have had many a last meal, and often I had many a last meal consecutive days in a row. Do you know what I am talking about? If I wasn't on a diet, then I was always getting ready to start a new diet. Before starting a new diet, I always gave myself permission to eat anything I wanted because I believed, in my head, that I would never again be able to eat the foods I liked, which I also considered as "bad" foods. Foods such as pizza, French fries, cheeseburgers, anything fried, bread, meat, rice, etc.

Of course, depending on the diet and its rules and regulations, I was still allowed to eat some of those foods. Often I would say, "Tomorrow I will start my diet," but then tomorrow would come, and I would have a reason why I would start my diet the following day.

I had many excuses such as, "It's my friend's birthday and we're going to dinner," or "Work is providing a free lunch," or "Oops, I accidentally ate too many fries, so I'll start tomorrow because today is shot."

The problem with thinking like this is that it actually creates more harm to your body. Usually you consume more unhealthy foods than you would if you were just choosing to eat what your body would like for that one specific meal. Also, if you are choosing to eat what your body requires, then there are no unhealthy foods.

Not only does it make you feel physically too full when you choose to eat like this, but you also feel guilty for overdoing it or for making those choices. You justify it and make yourself feel better by repeating the mantra that tomorrow you will start your diet. There is no tomorrow. Your present meal is the most important meal that you have because it is not in the past, and it is not in the future. Your present meal affects how you feel now.

I finally learned this after many years of following this same pattern. One day, I noticed that I didn't trust myself to start my diet tomorrow. I knew that I could not be trusted and I knew that when I meant to deprive myself, I usually ended up overdoing it beforehand. When I realized that I couldn't trust myself, it scared me. I didn't even trust myself! Now, I know it was because I was not connected with myself. I was separate from my relationship with my body. My spirit told me over and over, through the guilt, that what I was doing was hurting me, and my body told me when it felt too full, but I didn't listen. When I realized I didn't trust myself, I was finally beginning to wake up to a part of me. I began to analyze the pattern I had with food and dieting and it went like this:

- Dieting
- Losing weight
- Attaining my goal weight
- Eating what I wanted, and more, because I had reached the goal weight
- Gaining weight
- Getting ready to start a diet and having my last meals and feeling guilty

- Starting a new diet full of deprivation
- Attaining goal weight and returning to my old patterns

...and the cycle continued.

Eventually, I began to forgive myself for what I would do. Breaking a pattern requires forgiveness and grace.

If you made a choice and you feel guilty about it, forgive yourself, the choice has been made, it is done and you cannot undo it. There is no point in beating yourself up for something you would have chosen either way. However, having kindness and understanding with yourself will help break this cycle of guilt.

You may wonder why you make choices that create guilt within you. Instead of beating yourself up, ask yourself, "Why am I doing this? Is there something in my life that I need to have compassion on myself for?"

For example, when I quit smoking, and I was trying to get rid of my anxiety, I finally realized I had lost something that had always been there in my life and when I had that anxiety, I began saying, "Of course you're not feeling comfortable, you just lost this thing that was always there," and voila, with that acknowledgement, the anxiety went away.

If you make changes in your lifestyle with food and weight, you may feel uncomfortable at times, and that's okay. You have let go of something that was once always a go-to for you. Some people say you have to replace a habit with something else. I say, why do we need to replace it with anything? Instead, why don't we give ourselves grace for what's underneath there and acknowledge those feelings.

Is there something going on inside of you that if you acknowledged and allowed it to simply be, would give you ease?

There is no last meal. You will need to eat for the rest of your life in order to stay alive, but every meal does offer you the freedom to choose for that meal at that moment.

Next time the thought creeps in that you will eat something now because you won't have it after this last time, ask yourself if that's a true statement. Ask yourself if your body even wants that food right now. Ask your body what it would like to have.

What if every meal was a new opportunity for you to choose to love your body, to be kind to it and to honor it?

What if you never have to have a last meal again?

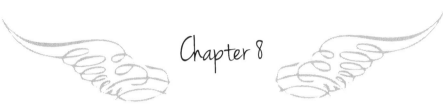

Chapter 8

What is a Normal Weight?

What is a normal weight? From my point of view, a normal weight is where your body naturally likes to be at without you fighting it. Throughout all of those years of dieting, starving, binging, and purging, I found that I would fight with my weight to be where I wanted it to be, but I also found that the times when I had given up the fight, it seemed that my body always went back on its own to a set point. For me, it's somewhere around a size 3/4/5. At this size, I feel good. I feel healthy and I look healthy. Some people would probably say that I am too skinny, while some would probably say I am just right, and others would probably say I need to lose some weight; everyone's got their point of view. Normal, or a "just right" weight, is where your body likes to be. It is not where you think it **should** be.

Norms change and differ from culture to culture, from country to country, from state to state, from city to city, from family to family, and even between circles of friends.

So what is truly your norm? When in your lifetime have you felt good about being in your body? Where does your body naturally set itself to when you stop trying to control it with food, starvation, and dieting? If you can't ever think of a time you felt good in your body, ask your body, "What is my norm?"

"Body, where would you feel good?"

"Body, what weight would you need to be at to feel at home?"

In fact, ask your body right now; let's do it. You do not need to worry about the answer right now. You may hear it in your head, you may get an answer in the form of a feeling, or you may receive knowingness in the form of a sign or some other gift. It may not happen right now, or tomorrow, but it will come to you when you are ready to know. So ask yourself:

"Body, what is MY normal?"

"Body, where do you feel good?"

"Body, where do you feel the most comfortable?"

"Body, what weight makes you feel at home?"

Do you see the kindness you are offering your body in your relationship with it? You are not telling it that it must be one way or another; instead you are including it in the relationship to make a decision.

I once had a boyfriend I loved with all of my heart. I mean, I LOVED this man. He liked to make most of the big decisions. This bothered me, and I began to wonder if I could spend the rest of my life with him in this way. We had made plans to move in together when my lease ended. One morning we were lying in bed, and he told me that when his parents retired they would move in with us. I was taken aback by this. I wasn't taken aback by the fact that he wanted to offer our future home as a place for his parents to permanently live (okay, maybe a little), I was taken aback because of the way he approached it. He never asked me how I felt about his parents living with us. He just stated this was the way things were going to be.

When we broke up, I wrote him a letter saying that I didn't know where I was in the relationship; he never considered my feelings or opinions at all when it came to the big stuff. You know, I probably would have not loved the idea of living with his parents, but I probably could have found a way of being okay with it if I had been offered a chance to be part of the decision-making in the relationship. That was it for our relationship. It was over. A relationship can't continue to be a relationship if only one person is calling all of the shots.

This is why it is not kind to tell your body it must be a certain weight or it must look a certain way. If you include your body in the relationship, your body will respond positively because your body loves you.

I loved that man; I wanted to work things out, but he wouldn't include me, so I had no choice but to walk away from that relationship. I knew that I deserved much more than what he was offering. I knew I deserved to be part of a relationship and included in the decision-making. I had a voice too. Your body has a voice as well, and it will let you know through pain, through putting on weight, heartburn, and other signs if it is happy or not. Listen to your body's voice. If you speak to your body and ask your body where it would like to be and what weight it is comfortable at, it will respond, honor you, and bless you. You will be pleasantly surprised.

How much more would you enjoy your life and your body if you included your body in the decision process?

Chapter 9

Your Body Relationship

I am not this hair,
I am not this skin.
I am the soul that lives within.
~Rumi

The relationship that you have with your body is the foundation for living a life free from weight and food obsession. Your relationship with your body is the key. When you use the tools and strategies, along with building a healthy relationship with your body, frustration and obsession fall away, and newfound freedom will become evident to you.

If your desire is to live a life free from worrying about your weight, the place to start is by understanding what a relationship with your body is and how to build one that is healthy, nurturing, and loving. You may be wondering what is a relationship with your body and how do you create a relationship with your body?

Everyone has a relationship with their body. A relationship with your body is just the same as you would have a relationship with anyone; your best friend, your mother, your father, your sister, your brother, your boyfriend, your girlfriend, your husband, your wife, your children, or yourself.

Not too many people are aware that they are currently in a relationship with their body. It is a give and a take between you and your body, between your spirit and your body, between your mind and your body. There is a relationship flow.

I too was completely unaware up until some years back when I began some transformational bodywork in the care of a gifted practitioner. It was there that I began connecting to my body and learning that I am spirit in my body and that I am not my body. I am NOT my body.

When I first realized that I was really free from thoughts about my weight and thoughts about food, and realized that I was just living my life, I asked myself, *What happened to make this occur? What things did I do to create this change?* There were a number of things that I noticed. I noticed that the tools and strategies that I learned throughout the years, that I was continuing to use, made a huge impact on my freedom. What made a huge shift within me was when I started connecting to my body, and I started building a relationship with my body. I began to understand that I am a spirit in my body, and my body and I are in a partnership.

This is an important concept to understand: You are NOT your body. You are a spirit within your body, but you are not your body. You and your body live together in a partnership.

Here is a small exercise to try out now:

Cover both of your eyes with your hands for a couple of minutes. Can you feel you inside your body? Can you feel your spirit inside your physical form? Just sit there for a couple of minutes and be with yourself in your body.

What did you notice?

Communicate with your body. Ask your body questions, such as, "Body, are you truly hungry?"

"Body, how can I honor you today?"

"Body, how would you like to move today?"

"Body, what food do you require today in order to feel healthy, vibrant, and at your best?"

What you are listening for is that little voice inside of you. For some of you, it may be a voice, for others of you it may be a feeling. It may take a little time and practice to trust the voice of your body, but the more you do it, the more you will know when your body is speaking to you and what it is saying to you. The more often you do it, the more your relationship with your body will grow. The more your relationship with your body grows, the more you will trust it. The more you trust your body, the more you will want to honor it. The more you honor your body, the more you will love it. The more you love your body, the kinder you will be to your body. The more you are kind to your body, the more your relationship will grow, and thus, *The Love Your Body Cycle* (page 21) continues.

Some of you may be thinking that talking to your body is the craziest thing you have ever heard. Take a moment and look at one of your hands. Do your best to leave any judgments out while you are doing this. Really look at your fingers. What do you call your fingers? Do you call them by your first name? No, you call them *my fingers*, just as you call anyone you have a relationship with, *my boyfriend, my girlfriend, my fiancé, my husband, my wife, my sister, my brother, my cousin,* but you are not them. You have a relationship with them, just as you do with your fingers. You are not your fingers, but you and your fingers work together. You have a thought, and that thought is fired through your nervous system and thus tells your fingers to do something such as to pick up your car keys, to answer the phone or to pick up the fork to eat.

It is the same for all of the other parts of your body; your legs, your feet and toes, your stomach, your back, your buttocks, your chest, your armpits, your arms and hands, your nose, your ears, your eyes, the list goes on. All parts of your body serve their purpose which is serving you. Take some time and think about what does each part of your body do to serve you? Are you grateful for what each part does? Or do you bash it and put it down because one part is too flabby or another is too big, or you wish you had the shape of someone else's body part?

How does your body serve you? What does your body do to serve you? Go ahead, make a list right now. What does your body do for you?

I'll give you a few examples of what my body does for me:

When I'm really hot, my body sweats to cool me down.
When I cut myself, my body heals the wound.
My back supports me so that I can walk.
My hands allow me to put food into my mouth to nourish myself.

My body eliminates waste.

My legs are strong, and they take me places.

My body responds to touch with joy and pleasure.

My tongue tastes food and lets me know if it is good or warns me if it is not.

My teeth break down the food I eat.

I can drive a car and get around places because I can see with my eyes.

My inner ears contribute to my body staying balanced.

I could make this list extensive because our bodies serve in a million ways.

When you can recognize what your body does for you, it will help you to understand the relationship that you have with your body. Once you understand the relationship that you have with your body, you will see things differently. Awareness changes everything. Once you are aware of something, you can never truly go back to where you were.

Did you make a list of what your body does for you?

As you are reading this book and learning all of these new tools and strategies, I want you to keep in the forefront of your mind that all of these tools work together with the relationship you have with your body. All of these tools are about being nurturing and kind.

To get started, I am going to ask you some questions about your relationships with people and I am going to ask that you write down your answers on a separate sheet of paper. You can write them out in bullet format, in sentences, in a paragraph. However you choose to write the answers to these questions is fine. This is very important to building the foundation of your relationship with your body, so please don't skip this part. You may need to set a little time aside to do this, to do this for you. Plan for about 30 minutes, give or take.

I truly believe that the connection and relationship you have with your body, and using the tools that I will teach you, is the key to freedom from weight obsession and the key to creating a beautiful body that you love, not just love with your heart, but physically you will love the way your body looks.

Alright, let's get started!

I want you to think about the people in your life that you have relationships with, and I want you to think about someone that you love, very, very much. It could be your lover, your best friend, your sister, whoever it is that you love dearly. Now think about the following questions.

How do you treat the person that you love?
- Do you speak to them kindly?
- Do you ask them how they are doing?
- Do you check in with them?
- Do you give them gifts?
- Do you randomly do kind things for them like buy them a coffee or flowers?
- How do you treat the person that you love?

Now write your thoughts down in response to: How do you treat the person you love?

How do you want the person that you love to treat you?
- Do you want them to consider you when making decisions?
- Do you want them to ask you how you are doing?
- Do you want to hear from them?
- Do you want them to call you?
- Do you want them to tell you that they love you and hug you and kiss you?

Now record your thoughts in response to: How do you want to be treated by the person that you love?

What would your ideal relationship be like with a lover?
- How would they treat you and how would you treat them?
- What would the communication between the two of you be like?
- How would they talk to you?
- How would you talk to them?

Write down what your ideal relationship with a lover would be like.

What is your relationship currently like with your body?
- Do you wake up in the morning, touch your body and tell it, "Body I love you and I am so grateful for you."
- Do you wake up in the morning and pinch your skin and check to see if you lost any weight from last night or if the cheeseburger that you had for dinner last night is sticking to your hips?
- Do you look in the mirror and say "OMG, you're so gross!"
- Do you withhold certain foods from your body?
- Do you punish your body with extra workouts for food that you have chosen to eat?
- Do you treat your body to massages?
- Do you nurture your body in any special way?

Take your time to write this out. Write out everything that you can think of that you know about how you treat your body, how you talk to your body, how you touch your body, how you look at your body, what you think about your body, what you feed your body, how you feel in your body, and anything else that you can think of that is related to you and your body.

What would you like your relationship to your body to be like?
- In a perfect world what would you like your relationship to be like with your body?
- Would you like to be happy with your body?
- Would you like to communicate with it?
- Would you like to not be obsessed with it?
- Would you like to trust your body?
- Would you like to speak kindly to it and about it?

Now, write out your thoughts about this last question. What would you like your relationship to your body to be like?

Next, I am going to ask you to go back through your lists and identify the similarities and differences between the relationships you have with people and the relationship you have with your body whether they be positive or negative.

As you are doing this, make note of what you notice. You can circle them; you can highlight them; you can star them; you can write them out; whatever works for you, just as long as you get the awareness of what those are.

- Are there any similarities between your relationship with the people you love and the relationship you have with your body?

- Now, go over your lists and notice where you have been kind to your body.

- Think about how your life would be if your relationship to your body were how you would like it to be.

- Next, review your lists and think about what are some ways that you can be kinder to your body? If you can't think of any or can't even imagine being kind to your body right now, no problem, in this book I will teach you how to be kind and loving to your body.

A relationship is between two things or two people. If you treat your partner or friend that you are in a relationship with, with kindness, how do they treat you back? With kindness, right?

If you are unkind to your partner, how do they respond? Usually, they will respond with unkindness as well.

If you ignore what your partner's needs are, what do they do? They try to get your attention, or they lash out in anger in some way.

Below are a few examples of how your body will respond when you are unkind to it.

If you choose to smoke, your body will eventually react with coughing or some other disease in the long term.

If you continue to purge your body of food by throwing up, it is possible you will wear out the lining in your esophagus, creating a disease.

A disease is not something that just happens to you for no reason; it is your body saying, "Hey! I am in dis-ease, notice me, pay attention, change something, something is not right!"

If you have indigestion from eating certain foods or too much of certain foods, your body is letting you know that it is not at ease. It is saying, "Hey, this hurts, stop, please!"

You don't just get indigestion for no reason.

Your body has its ways of communicating with you, just as people in a relationship will let you know when they are pissed off, hurt, or feeling loved.

Our bodies respond to the way they are treated and spoken to, just as people do.

Chapter 10

Trusting Your Body

I understand that letting go of control and trusting your body to do what it does can be a challenge and downright scary if you have always taken the reigns in your relationship with your body. Your body was made with the ability to function in balance and harmony, but it is what we do to it that throws it off of its balance.

People were not born with the need to battle their weight. This is a learned behavior from others around us and the media. Our bodies are quite capable of telling us what they need to eat, when they need to eat, and when they are finished eating. They are capable of digesting food properly and eliminating it as waste if we let them do their part and if we honor our bodies through what we put inside of them.

Just like in a relationship, if one person is doing all of the work, there is stress and frustration within that relationship, but if both people are listening to each other and honoring each other, the relationship flows. If one person is always nagging the other person to take out the garbage, clean the kitchen, water the plants, go pick up the dry cleaning, etc... the other person becomes resistant to doing anything, but if both people trust that the other person will take care of what they need to in the right time, then it gets done. If they ask each other what the other one needs, they can meet each other's needs and thus increase the communication and trust in their relationship.

Can you think back to a time when you trusted your body? Maybe it was recently, maybe it was last year, maybe it was five years ago, or maybe the last time you can remember trusting your body was when you were a child. Maybe you can't ever remember a time when you trusted your body. But, I can assure you, at one time you did, even if it was when you were an infant, and you cried when you were hungry. Your body let you know when it required food, and you then cried out for your parent or a caregiver to feed you and nourish your body. Your body let you know when it was hungry, and you made sure it was fed by letting others around you know that you were hungry. Your body trusted you to honor it and make sure it was fed, and you trusted it to let you know when it was hungry. You had a working relationship.

Over time, for whatever reasons, you and your body lost that mutual trust for each other. After many diets and unkind thoughts toward your body, your relationship became hurt, but it is possible to heal that relationship. It may require some blind faith from you and some blind trust in your body. But, what do you have to lose? If what you have been doing has brought you to a place of deep frustration with your body, your weight, and your thoughts, then what are your options? You can continue on the path you have been on or you can try something new.

Ask your body, "What would it take to build trust between us?"

and,

"What do you need from me in order to trust me?"

Remember, chances are you haven't been speaking very kindly to your body or treating it physically with love and kindness if you have been depriving yourself of food or overeating. Your body has to learn to trust you as well.

You may say, "I don't trust myself," and that's okay. If you are actively asking your body questions such as, "Body, are you truly hungry?" or, "Body, what would you like to eat?" you will find that it's not that hard to honor your body. When you experience this, you will begin to see that you can trust yourself to honor your body. You just never knew that you had a relationship with your body to honor.

Listening to your body will help you to create trust between you and your body. Ask it lots of questions. If you were rebuilding trust between you and a partner, what would you do to build that trust back up? Would you listen to that person? Would you check in with them more often? Would you tell them how much you care about them? Would you treat them extra well? It's the same with your body. Treat your body extra well in order to rebuild the trust and watch how your body responds. Your body will take care of you too.

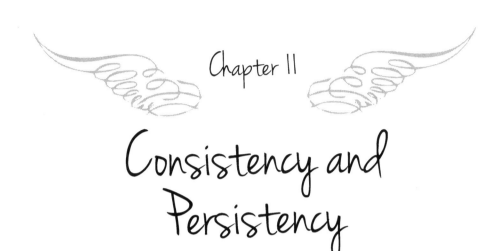

Chapter 11

Consistency and Persistency

*"The race is not always to the swift,
but to those who keep on running."*
Anonymous

I have a firm belief that success always comes if you continue to go in the direction of what you desire.

Too often when people diet and try to control their body, they eat something that makes them feel guilty, or they "fall off the wagon." The first thing they often do is say, "I blew my diet!" and then they continue to eat everything else they can get their hands on until they start their next diet, as if they made a mistake and now everything in between this mistake and the next diet doesn't count, but it does. It's abuse and neglect to the body, and the body will not react in kindness when treated this way.

Everything you stuff into your body between the time you "fall off the wagon" and you start your next diet, you will find your body has held on to and you will most likely see yourself as having even more weight to lose. This does not lead to weight loss, and this does not lead to having a relationship with your body that is kind and successful. However, this does contribute to yo-yo dieting and the rollercoaster that it is.

When I eat something that doesn't sit well with me, or when I think I haven't really been doing a good job of listening to what my body wants to eat, I don't head to the fridge or the drive-thru. I pick up exactly where I am, and I make my choices based on where I am. This is kindness, and this is forgiveness, and this is grace. We may not be able to undo the past, but we can always choose for ourselves in this present moment.

The first personal trainer that I ever had, back when I was 18 years old, told me that the key to having an "in shape" body was to be consistent with working out. Yo-yo dieting is not consistent; binging and purging is not consistent. Well, they are consistent at not being consistent and will result in you not loving your body.

So, when you make a choice that you are not thrilled about, or when you have "fallen off the wagon," climb right back on that wagon. Don't wait for Monday or next week, immediately decide to make choices that result in you being kind to your body, and if you don't know what that is, ask your body, "Body, what can I do right now to be kind to you? Body, what can I choose right now that would make you feel at peace?"

And remember that you don't ever have to try to figure out what the answers are. The answers will come. Your body will let you know, you just have to be quiet, patient, and listen.

When you are consistent with asking your body how it would like to move and what it would it like to eat, and then consistent with listening to it, then you will most likely begin to notice the weight loss you have been trying to achieve for so long, happen naturally. But please don't make weight loss the reason you ask your body questions, because then you will be focusing on the weight again, and as long as you focus on the weight, the weight will be an issue.

Chapter 12

Does Your Body Trust You?

If you are reading this because you are a yo-yo dieter, obsessed with food or obsessed with your weight, then you already know that you don't trust your body. Take a moment to look at your track record and all of the ways you have withheld nourishment from your body, withheld pleasure, kept your body inside the house at times because you were ashamed of it or embarrassed of it, told it unkind words, or forcefully purged food from your body.

In order to rebuild and repair the trust in the relationship with your body, it may require some extra loving care and attention from you.

It occurred to me one day as I was thinking about how my body used to react to my inconsistent dieting, binging and purging, starvation, and unkind words, what if my body was responding to the way I treated it? There were times when I would work out 2 hours a day, eat no carbohydrates, and not lose a pound after weeks of this regime, leaving me baffled.

After many years of confusing my body with different ways of eating, it began to happen that my sense of fullness was very confused or shut off. I could not predict if I was still hungry, just right, or full because the sensation of fullness would hit me 1, 2, or 3 hours later. It was the most bizarre thing. I could eat a very tiny amount, like 1/2 a sandwich, and two hours later I would be stuffed. It made no sense to me. I was very frustrated and unsure of what I could eat and how much I could eat.

I never got the message my body was sending me until years later. My body was telling me that it knew that I didn't trust it, and it was giving me the same message back by literally becoming what I could not trust. I could not trust how my body would react to any amount of food I put in it. It was trying to get my attention in this way.

Does your body trust you?

Should your body trust you?

Is your body sending you messages?

If so, what kinds of messages and what do you do when you receive messages from your body?

Chapter 13

Nothing to Fix

When I first quit smoking, I was not worried about my weight. I felt very strong and very solid with where I was with my relationship with my body. Within a few days of quitting smoking, my then loose shorts became tight on me. I was okay with that and chalked it up to water weight, which is natural when one quits smoking. I was also happy to be doing something kind for my body, such as quitting smoking.

I had done a lot of research on smoking and the effects it has on the body. I continued to come across stories and research about how people gain weight when they quit. For just a short while, I began checking my body in the mirror. Thoughts began to stir within me that I should watch what I am eating since I quit smoking. Of course, I noticed this right away and reminded myself that these were not acts of kindness. I was chewing a lot of gum because I had all of this nervous and uncomfortable energy since I quit smoking, and while I didn't feel like eating for the nervousness, I didn't know what to do with that energy and I wanted to get rid of it.

Then one day, I was watching a video on the internet that someone had made when he said, "What if there is nothing to fix?" and my whole body went, "Ahhhhhh."

I rewound the video and replayed it, "What if there is nothing to fix?"

Once again, my body went, "Ahhhhh. Yes! That's it!"

He continued, "What if everything is just a message from your body?"

That's when it hit me; I had been ignoring the messages from my body. Even after everything I knew about listening to my body, I was still missing what it was trying to tell me. All of that nervous tension and uncomfortableness that I had been feeling was my body's way of trying to get my attention. I did not need to fix my uncomfortableness. I needed to acknowledge it, to go towards it, to pet it like an animal with love, to hold it and cradle it like a newborn baby.

You see, when I quit smoking, I lost a relationship that was constant in my life for many, many years. It may not have been a healthy relationship, but it was a relationship. It was always there with me to celebrate the good times. It was there with me in the sad times, when I was bored, when I was lonely, and well, it was just always there. When I let this relationship go, even though I wanted to and it was my choice all the way, I was left with a sense of not knowing how to cope in this world, how to be, how to deal with the hard times and how to enjoy the good times, so I felt very uncomfortable. I continued to try to get rid of this uncomfortable feeling. I prayed, I meditated, I tried yoga; I moved my body more, but it only became greater and louder. I was beginning to feel that I was fighting with myself, and that is such the opposite of what I practice.

When I watched this video, it hit me. Bam! I wasn't listening to myself! I wasn't listening to my body. Instead, I was treating myself harshly and without grace and meanwhile I had just lost a very large relationship in my life. I was grieving, but not allowing myself to grieve freely with permission.

As soon as I had that revelation, everything changed. I couldn't believe how unkind I had been to myself about feeling so uneasy in my skin. I would never say to a friend of mine that recently got out of a relationship, "What can you do to get rid of what you are feeling?"

No, I would say, "It's okay that you are feeling this way, of course, you are feeling this way. You spent a huge part of your life in this relationship. Of course, it's going to feel uncomfortable at times."

No joke, immediately after that, the uneasiness cleared up as I allowed myself to recognize that I was grieving, grieving the loss of my relationship to a cigarette, and allowed myself to acknowledge that, at times, I did not feel like myself without smoking.

It's interesting how once I said to myself, *You know what? Oh my gosh, I have not given myself grace for the loss of this relationship.* It's interesting how the next morning everything changed. I was able to focus on where I was and not on the anxiety that I was trying to fight. Instead of trying to fight the anxiety, I went towards it saying, "This is okay."

Then, the anxiety went away on its own because I acknowledged it and its purpose. I acknowledged how it could be helpful, and I acknowledged its life, and then with that acknowledgment, its job was served, its purpose was served, it didn't need to continue.

My body was sending me a message in the form of anxiety that I needed to pay attention to something, instead of trying to fix it. Usually, when we pay attention and acknowledge without trying to fix something that something we were trying to fix in the first place, goes away on its own.

What if there is nothing about your body that you need to fix? What if instead you acknowledged the messages your body is sending you? And if you are unclear about what those messages are, ask your body, "Body, will you please show me what you want me to be aware of in a way that is clear to me?" and then drop it.

You do not need to figure out what the messages are. Your body will let you know, in a way that is clear to you, because you asked, because you are communicating with your body, and because you are engaged in a relationship with your body.

When I first started a particular type of bodywork, I had tightness in my shoulders sometimes that was very uncomfortable. The discomfort, I believe, was due to stress. When I told my caregiver, he said, "Tell that part of your body that you are aware that it is working on getting a message through to you, just acknowledge it."

Nine out of ten times the tightness would go away. There wasn't even anything I had to figure out or a message that I needed to consciously *get*, but just acknowledging that part of my body made the unease become at ease.

The next time you are experiencing unease, remember that there is nothing to fix, but instead acknowledge whatever it is that is coming up. Be present with it and allow it to be whatever it is.

Some questions you can ask in order to help yourself acknowledge and be present when uncomfortable feelings arise are:

Body, what are you trying to tell me?

Body, what message are you sending me that I am not aware of?

Will you make me aware in a way that feels more comfortable?

Is there a place and a space where I can give myself grace right now that I have not seen?

What part of me needs to be acknowledged and loved right now?

What if there is nothing to fix?

Chapter 14

Honor Yourself

The spirit wants to be free. Your spirit and my spirit desire choice. When we deny our spirit the honor of choosing, we create conflict within ourselves. It is that voice of conflict that chatters away in our head making us feel guilty and uneasy.

My father always said, "You are a free spirit and you have free will, you can choose for you; no one can make you do anything."

So, why do we take the choice away from our spirit and our body and restrict what it can or cannot eat?

We all have different parts of us that all serve a purpose and have a will. I believe that all of these parts work together, and when each part is honored, we can find ourselves at peace. One of these parts is the physical body that we are in, the second part is our mind, our mind that thinks and makes decisions, and the third is our spirit, the part of us that feels and connects with others, the part of us that loves.

The moment you start thinking about what you should or shouldn't do, your body starts reacting. Are you aware of how your body reacts? For me, I feel tense, I feel anxious, and my neck will get tight. I start feeling like I am wrong, like I am making mistakes, like I am messing things up. I then become unhappy, questioning myself, my judgments and my choices. My spirit is not at ease when my mind starts thinking about things I should do, instead of honoring my spirit and following what I would like to do or what feels right or light.

One morning in Rome, during the summer of 2012, I woke up and asked myself, "What would you like to do to honor yourself today?"

I gave myself permission to do anything that I really wanted to do, and nothing that I should do, unless I really wanted to do that. That day was one of the best days of my life.

What does it mean to honor yourself?

Honoring you means taking care of you. It means treating yourself like you are special and important, because you are. It means every day doing something for yourself that you enjoy, and not that you have to do. I know that we live in a busy world, and most of us are busy people. I get that. I get that there are a ton of things we feel we must do, but if you can wake up each day and just ask, "If I could do one thing to honor me today, what would it be?" and then do it, you will find yourself in a newfound state of happiness, because your spirit will be so honored.

Honoring you doesn't have to take hours, it may be as simple as taking 20 minutes to sit down and read a chapter from a book that you have been putting off, or calling a friend, or signing up for a class you've been wanting to take, or going to the mall to buy yourself the shirt you saw in an advertisement, or just going for a walk in the park, or it may just be sitting quietly in the bathroom away from everyone and everything for 5 minutes to take some time and peace to yourself. Honoring you is you giving yourself kindness and taking action on fulfilling your needs.

When you have a free day, or if you choose to find time to give yourself a free day, ask yourself on that day, "What can I do to honor myself today?" and then do it.

You will have one of the best days of your life. You will notice so many gifts that pop up into your universe that you will be amazed and want to have more days where you just honor yourself. I have met incredible people in different places that are still in my life today because I took a day to honor myself. Miracles happen when you honor yourself, because you step into a space of openness where you are not concerned about the must-dos and you just follow the energy.

When you honor your body, magic happens too. It's as simple as asking each morning, "Body, if there was one thing that I could do today to honor you, what would it be?" or "Body, how can I honor you today?"

Your body may say it wants a massage, or it wants a bath, or it wants to dance, or it wants to sleep, or it wants to be wrapped up in a blanket sitting in front of the TV, or it may just want you to take your hand and place it over your heart and feel your own heart beating.

When you ask your body, and then listen and respond, you strengthen the relationship with your body and your connection with your body. This connection will affect every other aspect of your life because you will feel good about you and about being in your body.

I know that most of us have to work and have commitments such as a spouse or children, but ask yourself every day, "What can I do to honor myself today?"

You are totally worth it and deserving of it. Another gift from all of this is if your children see and hear you honoring yourself, they will learn to honor themselves too.

Grab a pen and some paper and jot down your answers to the following questions:

Where in your life have you not been honoring you?

How have you not been honoring your body?

What things or people are you making more important than you?

Where in your life can you honor you?

How can you honor your body?

If you can, rearrange your schedule for just one day so that you can take an entire day just to honor you. Let me know what happens. I'd love to hear about the magic that shows up in your life. Seriously! Connect with me through the book club. You can go to www.lemuelachristina. com to join and it's free.

In my journey through life, I have learned that if you do not honor yourself, you cannot honor someone else. In honoring yourself and loving yourself, you can honor someone else and love them more because you will have more to give them. So honor you, honor your spirit, and the rest will follow. You will have so much more to give to others and to all the other aspects of your life, your career, your relationships, your friendships, and anything else that is important to you.

What magic will show up in your life when you begin to honor yourself and to honor your body?

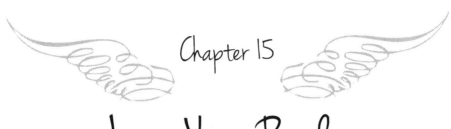

Chapter 15

Love Your Body

Loving your body has many meanings. It means being kind to your body, communicating with your body, and listening to it. It means honoring it, giving it what it needs, and taking care of it. When you have a healthy relationship with your body and communicate effectively with your body, your body takes on the shape and form of a body that you love.

It is through loving and nurturing your body that you will have the beautiful body you have always wanted. Does it sound too good to be true? Well, it's true, and it only requires you choosing it. When you yo-yo diet, obsess about your weight, and beat yourself up for the way you look, your body responds exactly to that and gives you exactly what you tell it.

When we connect with our bodies in a loving way, things begin to change in our world. Everyday routines happen with more ease, we are more at peace, we respond to people and life with more joy, and people gravitate to our being more. Why? Because when we connect with our body, our body, mind and spirit can be together in harmony instead of separated.

One big way that you can love your body is by communicating with it, and there are many ways that you can do that. You may already practice many of these forms of communication, but doing these things with the intent to connect and love your body, will bring you rewards that you were never aware of before.

Getting a Massage

Massage is direct attention on the body that involves caring for it and nurturing it in a slow, quiet, and present way. Some people have found that massage has given them benefits such as stress relief, relief from insomnia related to stress, relief from headaches, and some have even found their digestion improving. Massage is also a great way to cleanse the body of toxins.

Our bodies love touch and respond to touch.

I love massages because I get to just lay there and do nothing while my body is totally pampered and loved. I love the way it feels to focus on that area that is being touched. Massage is a great way to let go of the day, and to let your mind just be.

Moving Your Body

Yoga, walking, and playing a sport are all examples of ways that you can move your body. When you are moving your body, be aware of what it feels like to be in your body, to be the spirit that you are inside of this beautiful gift you have called a body. Praise it for what it can do.

I speak more about moving your body in the chapter *Move Your Body*.

Meditating

There are a plethora of benefits to meditating, and it can be done anywhere, with or without music, sitting or lying down. There are tons of classes out there, and you can also find many guided meditations either for purchase or for free online.

Checking in with Your Body

You can check in with your body at any time. I prefer first thing in the morning because it is quiet, and it is a good time for me to connect with my body before I get up to start the day.

When I check in with my body, I find a quiet place to lay down on my back, but if I am not in a situation to find a quiet place and I feel that

I need to check in, then I just find a place to sit. With my eyes closed I take both of my hands and place them on any part of my body. Then with my mouth closed, I inhale through my nose and exhale out of my mouth, while being present in the area where my hands are resting. I do that a few times and then move to another area of my body and re-peat. I repeat the breathing and being present with that part of my body. Whenever my hands are on these different places on my body, I am making a nice warm, friendly contact with my body. In a sense, I am holding that part of myself. I am just acknowledging my body and feel-ing my spirit inside of my body. I am being present, and still and quiet. That's all. It's that simple.

Asking Your Body Questions

Usually, in the morning, when I am checking in, I will also ask my body some questions or let it know what I am grateful for. Here are some examples of questions I ask my body:

"Body, what can I do to honor you today?"

"Body, what can I do be kind to you today?"

"Body, what would you like to receive today?"

"Body, how would you like to move today?"

"Body, what would you like to wear today?"

You can ask your body whatever feels right to you. The answer will come in a knowing, a feeling, a picture in your mind, or a thought of something that when you think about it, feels nice and light.

During the day if you are feeling out of sorts or you are feeling down, stressed, anxious, or if you have a headache or some kind of pain or unease in your body, you can ask it a question. Here are a few examples of questions I have used when I have felt unease in my body:

"Body, what do you need right now?"

"Body, what do you need from me right now?"

"Body, what do you want me to know?"

"Body, what is it that you are telling me that I am not getting?"

Once again, the answer will come to you in the form of a knowing, or a sense, or a feeling, and sometimes there is no answer that comes to you, but you realize later that the unease is gone. Often, just by acknowl-edging the unease in your body, the unease dissipates.

Sometimes our bodies just need us to acknowledge them, and they send us a physical message in order to get us to do that, and once we acknowledge the message instead of fighting it, the unease and discomfort go away. Just as in a relationship, your partner wants to be heard, and you want to be heard by your partner, and once you are heard, you stop nagging or complaining about that which is bothering you.

Gratitude Touch

You can thank your body at any time; when you are driving, when you are walking to your car, or first thing in the morning after you hit the snooze button. You can put your hand on any part of your body that you would like to thank and express your gratitude towards it. When you rest your hand on any part of your body that you are about to thank, observe with your mind's eye, that part of your body first. That's a really good way to connect with it, to feel it, and to bring up the feeling of gratitude.

You can put your hands on your legs. Observe your legs with your mind's eye. What a gift they are! Think about what they do for you and thank your legs. For example, "Thank you, legs, for being strong enough to carry me every day and everywhere that I go."

"Thank you for the gift of movement."

You can move your hands onto your stomach, "Thank you stomach for having the awareness of what is enough for me and for digesting my food every day. Thank you for the intuition you lead me with."

"Thank you intestines for all that you do and for eliminating waste from my body."

You can move your hands to your eyes, "Thank you, eyes, for giving me the blessing to see the world."

Covering your ears, "Thank you ears that I can hear music and the voices of people."

Touching your mouth, "Thank you mouth for the ability to talk and to taste."

Holding your hands, "Thank you fingers and hands for the gift it is to be able to hold someone else's hand, to pick up this book to read, to be able to hold a fork."

Hugging yourself, "Thank you, arms, for the gift of being able to hug and express love."

With both hands on your chest, "Thank you, chest, for my breasts and for being a part of my body that is strong."

Hands on your back, "Thank you, back, for supporting my entire body."

Hands on your buttocks, "Thank you bootie for your support, a place to sit, and for how much fun you are to take dancing!"

Hands on your feet, "Thank you, feet, for being strong, supporting the weight of this body and for taking me places."

You get the idea. You can thank any and every part of your body in any way that you want to, even your hair!!! Those are just some specific examples I use, but, of course, you know what you are grateful for specifically for your body. If you feel that you are not grateful because you are bitter towards your body, then give your body thanks anyway, over time your heart will begin to be open to being genuinely grateful towards your body. If you can't put your hand on your body, then you can just thank the different parts of your body. Gratitude is like a magic wand.

Our bodies love to be touched and thanked. Our bodies love hugs, to be held, or when someone puts a kind hand on our arm, so why not extend the gift of touch to your own body? Your body will love it.

Having a Conversation with Your Body

Having a conversation with your body can include speaking to it and asking it questions. I have had conversations where I have apologized to my body for a choice that I made that was not kind. It doesn't always have to do with food. It could be that I stayed up way too late and then the next day my body was sluggish and unmotivated, my spirit was unsatisfied, and I just felt yucky and cranky overall. When I stay up too late, and do not get the 8-9 hours of sleep per night that my body likes, my body will let me know the next day how unhappy it is. I'm sure you have experienced this before at some time.

You can talk to your body anytime for any reason, to let it know how much you love it, how grateful you are to it, or if you feel the need to apologize, or you simply want to ask it a question. Your body loves to be in communication with you. Your body is ALIVE, so don't ignore it.

The Power of Being Grateful for Your Body

I'm going to tell a little story about the magic of gratitude and how our thoughts and feelings affect the way our body responds.

One of my very good friends was in a motorcycle accident in Rome, Italy, and he was very angry at the girl who made a wrong move and hit him. He was angry that he was in pain with a swollen hand, a swollen knee, and his back was beginning to hurt too. When I asked him how he was doing, he said that he was worried because he was still in pain.

I asked, "How long ago was the accident, 6 days?"

He replied that he was worried about his knee because it was still hurting after 6 days. I told him his body was still in the early stages of healing and then I told him, "Speak to your body, literally, thank it for all that it does for you and for all of the healing it has done already. Show your body gratitude, and it will recover even quicker. Your body is a living organism, and you are a spirit in your body, but you are not your body."

He then replied, "I'll try."

I said, "Think about what it is like when you are in a relationship with someone, how do they respond to your kindness and love? They love you back. If you give in a relationship, the other person wants to give back to you. This is the same with the relationship that you have with your body."

He said, "Mmmmmm… my last relationship was… uhm, I don't remember, hahaha."

"My friend, yes, well then think of any relationship… a friend, for example. When someone does something for you, let's say they treat you to a nice dinner, don't you want to do something nice back for them?" I responded.

And with that he replied, "Yes, of course."

I told him, "It is the same here. Most people are not connected to their body and when they begin to connect with their body, recognize their relationship, and make decisions and choices to honor their body, and speak to their body and listen to what their body is telling them, incredible things happen with their body such as healing, reduced stress, and weight loss. I know this, I have lived it."

"Remember, I told you that I am not connected," he said.

"It just takes awareness, but you can start whenever you want, and maybe with gratitude is a good place to start. I read somewhere that a person cannot be unhappy and express gratitude at the same time," I finished.

He thanked me, and our conversation came to a close.

We always have the choice to choose for us, and we are always choosing something. Some choices come with more effort than others because they are brand new to our world.

When you are not used to being grateful or not used to moving your body, or not used to meditating or checking in, it can take some effort to get started. But, aren't you worth it? Isn't your spirit worth it? Isn't your body worth it? Isn't the balance of you worth it? Don't you deserve to be the best you that you can be for you?

I tell that story of my conversation with my friend because you may have noticed he had a little resistance to what I had to say. My friend and I have had a few conversations about him connecting with himself, but to just converse doesn't make a change. One must rise to action in order to create change.

I also was in my own motorcycle accident the previous year in Rome when I went there for the summer. After the accident I had a bruise on my left tailbone about the size of a baseball. It turned a very deep shade of purple and black. I was in a lot of discomfort the first few days, but what happened to my discomfort and bruise in just a short period of time was a miracle. I believe the miracle occurred in response to my choices and my actions.

Because of my relationship with my body and my awareness of it, within minutes after the accident, once the ambulance had arrived and the paramedics were asking me if I wanted to go to the hospital, my first thought was, *I need to get a massage.* I was in tune enough to know what my body needed in order to begin healing itself. Within a couple of hours after the accident, I went and sought out a gentle Thai massage. I had remembered seeing a Thai massage parlor just the day before in my neighborhood in Trastevere.

Little did I know that seeing that place would be such a gift to me in my immediate future. I had a massage every day for the first few days, and then I tapered off to every other day, twice a week, and then once a week for a two month period. Was it costly? Yes, I took a chunk of money from my savings for it, but my body was worth it.

After that accident, my mind was more connected to God than I think it ever has been. I was in a constant state of gratitude. I was incredibly grateful to be alive! To be alive! To have my legs and my arms! My face was untouched. Even in my sleep I was thanking God for my life and my body. I also found a network chiropractor in Rome. I was so fortunate for this, and I saw him the first week three times. This type of work is also referred to as Network Spinal Analysis (NSA), and the care that is given involves reorganizational healing. I LOVE this work!

After a week of NSA, my bruise that was VERY there and VERY dark had vanished! It went from that deep dark to a kind of greenish-yellow and then one morning I turned to look in the mirror at it, and it was gone. I thought I was crazy. It had only been 7 days since the accident. What happened to the bruise? When I went in for my 4th visit, I told my care provider about this, and he said, "It's incredible, your body is like you never were even in a motorcycle accident."

I told him something magical happened between the care I received in his office, the Thai massages, and the gratitude that was overflowing within me. The intense discomfort that I had initially felt in my lower back was gone. It had completely vanished. I never had any residual pain from that accident ever.

I chose to nurture my body and to take care of my body. I was so gentle and kind to it. My loved one, my body, was worth me giving it the rest it needed. It was worth me spending the money on gentle massages and NSA. My body was worth me being grateful that I had it. The pain was the pain. Instead of resisting the pain, I felt it and was grateful that I had all of my parts to feel that pain. With all of these things put together, my body healed in record time.

I also want to note that when our bodies give us messages and when we receive and acknowledge the messages, the pain or the sensation or the physical change or whatever it is, often diminishes or leaves. In my case, I was at a point in my life where I wasn't happy or unhappy. I was just kind of floating by, and it was the reason I chose to move to another country for the summer. I knew I needed a wake up, and boy did I receive that message with a lightning bolt! I also did not mention how that same morning, about 20 minutes before the accident, I had fallen down half a flight of stairs in my apartment building. I ignored it. I did not ask, "What's the message in this? Body, why did you trip and fall? What are trying to tell me?"

I did not ask any of those questions. Instead, I went back to my apartment popped some ibuprofen and then went on my way to meet my friend who was picking me up on the motorcycle.

So, I finally got the message the universe was sending me. It was telling me to wake up to my life and be grateful for what I had, most importantly my life. I truly believe that my gratitude healed me so quickly because my body responded to all of those thoughts of gratefulness and was wrapped in love as I was so very, very grateful for my body.

If you express gratitude towards your body and towards your life in every way that you can, you will see gifts show up in your life that you would have never imagined possible.

Gratitude heals!

Listening

Stories on how to listen to your body are woven throughout this book, just like when I healed from my motorcycle accident. The art of listening to your body, requires you to pay attention. The more you are in tune to your knowing, the more you will begin to trust it and be able to respond to it right away. A great place to start if you feel disconnected from your body is by taking some time to just be with it and observe it. This is the same in a relationship with a person. If you are feeling disconnected from someone, spend time with them, listen to them, and you will rebuild the disconnection and heal your relationship.

Being still and just observing your body is a powerful way that you can connect with your body. Just lying there and being aware of any sensations, ticks, movements of energy, or energy swirling or circulating in a particular part of your body, or buzzing, or whatever feeling or sensation that you are aware of, is a great way to connect and listen to it. There is nothing to do, but to just be and acknowledge what you are feeling.

Sometimes, I will feel a lot of energy in one area of my body, and then I will just ask it, "Energy where would you like to go?"

"How would you like to be?"

Or, I will just acknowledge it and say, "Hello," to it. Literally.

You can even welcome it and tell it, "You are safe to be here and to be whatever you need to be."

You can ask your body, "Will you help me to hear you when you are sending me messages?

"Will you make me more aware of what you are telling me?"

Listening to your body is an art, and the more you practice this art, the more you will become aware of what you know, and the more you become aware, the more you can honor yourself and your body.

Kindness

One way to build a strong relationship with your body is to be kind to it. Kindness comes in many forms; such as how you treat your body, how you speak to it, and what and how you feed it. When you communicate kindly with your body, you build trust. Thank your body for all of the gifts it gives you and for all of the ways it serves you. Tell your body you love it, every day, and throughout the day. Ask your body what it would like to eat. Sit down with your food, eat slowly, and enjoy each bite. You deserve not to be rushed when eating. Ask your body how you can honor it today. Would it like a hot bath, a massage, to go for a walk, a few minutes of quiet and rest, to be touched and thanked? When you bless your body with kindness, your body will bless you back.

Getting a massage, moving my body, checking in, asking questions, talking, listening, and being grateful are just some ways that I communicate with my body that I have found are effective, have strengthened my relationship with my body, and given me more peace within myself.

Will you choose to love your body and communicate with your body?

How will you love your body?

How will you communicate with it?

For today, what do you choose to do to communicate with your body that you love it?

Chapter 16

Believe in What You Eat

Years ago, I began reading a book about inflammation in the body. I had picked this book up because my nose was constantly stuffed, and I still had swollen joints on occasion. Someone had recommended the book to me.

I took many of the suggestions in the book and pretty much cut out everything from my diet except vegetables and nuts. I got very creative with making soups, spaghetti squash, and any other creative meal I could make with vegetables. I felt healthy, energetic, and my inflammation dissipated. Of course, I lost weight as a result. My focus wasn't on losing weight. My focus was on my health, and weight loss was a side effect.

In the long run, I couldn't stick to that for longer than a few weeks as I was too hungry all the time. I had to find more foods that I believed were good for me to eat. I began adding foods back in over the weeks and months; organic cheese, rice, whole grains, and organic eggs for example. I was eating for my health and not for my weight.

I only bought organic food, and I did not eat red meat or chicken. I want to be clear here, while I still do not eat red meat or chicken in general, it is not a rule I follow, and in the past few years I have had myself a handful of juicy organic cheeseburgers cooked at home on the grill when my body was really craving one, not when I was craving a cheeseburger because I smelt it in the air coming from a restaurant I was passing by, but because my body was telling me it needed something from it. I do not consider myself a vegetarian, but I generally don't eat meat because of the way my body responds to it if I eat it consistently.

In general, my body does not respond well to hormones. If I eat foods on a regular basis such as red meat and chicken which have their own hormones and then are injected with additional hormones, my joints will swell. For me it's the same with the birth control pill, so I don't take that either. I don't eat meat because my body does not like it due to its sensitivity to hormones.

Once again, developing a relationship with your body will guide you in knowing what it likes. For years, my swollen joints were telling me that my body did not like something that I was putting in it. I knew that something was not at ease in my body. I went to the doctors and had tests run, but they couldn't figure it out.

Once, when I had just turned 30 years old, every joint in my body swelled up so bad that I could barely move, and the pain was excruciating. After three days of this, I was very scared. I knew that something was not right. I went to the emergency room in the middle of the night. It was my first time ever being a patient in a hospital. I was scared, and I was alone. The nurse gave me some Percocet for the pain and, if I remember correctly, I was given 800mg of ibuprofen to take every 6 hours.

They ran some tests, and the doctor said, "I don't want to scare you, but I think you may have Lupus."

I immediately started crying and freaking out that I had Lupus. I didn't even know what exactly it was, but I had heard of it and it scared me immensely. He told me that they would have the results in a couple of days from my blood test, and he would get back to me.

A few days passed, and I got a call, I did not have Lupus. What a relief! The doctor then told me that I should go see a specialist for more tests, so I went. The specialist couldn't come up with anything from his test results either.

I suggested to the specialist that I thought it was caused by hormones because I had just recently, in the last year, gotten off of the birth control pill and my chronic swollen shoulder joints were not chronically swollen anymore. He said that it couldn't possibly be hormonally related. So

I left his office with no medical answers, but an inkling that I was right about the hormones.

For me, stress can also swell my joints. Stress also affects hormones. At the time when I went to the emergency room for my whole body swelling, I was under a tremendous amount of stress at work, so I think that's what caused my body to react in such a way. It was giving me a sign, a big, huge warning sign that I needed to change something, and guess who knew my body? Guess who knew what had caused my body to go into a state of swollen shut down? I did. At least I believe I did, so I began taking more time for myself, meditating, and being aware of the level of my stress and how I was reacting to situations in my life.

My point is our bodies tell us. We just have to be willing to listen. If it sounds too simple, that is because it really is that simple.

I always tell my clients to know what they are eating and putting into their mouth and thus their body.

It is important for you to educate yourself. Learn about the different types of foods that are out there, such as organic versus natural. Is your food genetically modified? Is your food sprayed down with pesticides? If you drink diet sodas, do you know how the aspartame in them affects your body?

If you eat diet foods, educate yourself on what types of substitute sugars are going into those products and how they affect your weight and your health. Look at your labels and research some of those ingredients that you cannot pronounce and then decide if that product is something that honors your relationship with your body or if it hinders it. There are certain additives that cause migraines. Educate yourself, and you will create a belief system and begin to eat for the health of your body and not for the size of your body. Incredibly enough, when you begin eating for your health, weight loss is a natural side effect.

Get straight on your beliefs about food. Chances are you know very well what your body likes to eat and doesn't like to eat. You are probably very familiar with the messages your body sends you after you eat your meals; you just may not have been consciously aware of them. If you are receiving messages of heartburn, your body is letting you know that it does not like the food that caused the heartburn or perhaps how much food was taken in. If you are receiving messages of anxiety after having a drink with caffeine, your body does not like caffeine, so have your coffee decaffeinated if you must still have coffee. If, after you start eating one piece of pizza, you can't stop until you're grotesquely full; this is your body saying it does not like pizza because it has an allergy to some ingredient in that food that creates an addictive response.

When you honor your body, your body honors you. When you are kind to your body, your body is kind to you. When you take care of your body, your body takes care of you.

Chapter 17

Sugar

My body doesn't like processed sugar. I know because when I eat it, I can't stop. I crave more, and I feel tired from it. I'll give you an example of one of my many out of control experiences that I have had with processed sugar. I used to teach third grade in an outdoor mobile classroom that had two classrooms connected by a door in the middle. My teammate, who is also one of my best friends, was in her room one day during our planning period. I was craving some chocolate, so I asked her if she had any. She handed me a bag filled with miniature sized peanut butter cups. I took two and handed the bag back to her. I ate them, sat down at my desk to get back to planning, and all I could think about was that I just wanted one more. So I went back to my teammates room, "Steph, can I have just one more?"

"Sure," she replied, so I took two.

I did this a couple of more times until she said, "Do you want me to hide the bag in my car?"

I couldn't stop. I said, "Yes, but let me just have one more!"

I have countless stories and memories of me not being able to put processed chocolate down, or not being able to have just one, two, or three pieces of cake or of me eating one cookie after another, after another, after another, until finally I had to stop because I felt my stomach was going to burst.

My belief is that I have an allergy to processed sugar. One of the definitions of an allergy from *Thefreedictionary.com*, says that an allergy is *a hypersensitivity to a substance that causes the body to react to any contact with that substance.* My body reacts to processed sugar if I eat it on a daily basis, specifically processed chocolate with processed sugar. My body becomes addicted to it if I eat it on a daily basis. I think about it, and then I have to have it, and when I have it, I cannot stop until I'm disgustingly full.

Like meat and chicken, I have had little pieces of dessert a handful of times over the past few years. There have been two Thanksgivings where I have had a tiny sliver of my brother-in-law's pumpkin pie. Once, last summer in Italy, I bought a gelato, took a couple of licks and threw it out because it was so sweet.

In my last year as an elementary teacher in Westminster, Colorado, I had a sleepover with my two best teacher friends and there was a tub of chocolate ice cream in the freezer. They were going to have some and I thought, *I'm solid; I can have a bowl of that ice cream.* And I did. I had a bowl, and then I had another and another, and I may have even had another. Whatever happened, I finished it off, and when I finished it, I had to laugh at what had just happened. I lost control when I had processed sugar and chocolate, because my allergy never went away.

I never bashed myself for that incident. Instead, I was grateful that it had happened. It was a reminder to me that I cannot eat processed sugar and chocolate without losing control. So I let it go. I was grateful that instead of beating myself up or feeling guilty for it, I could just look at it as a learning experience and view it as a reminder of what is true for me and move on with my life.

People have told me that I am depriving myself, or I don't know what I am missing. I will gladly not have dessert for the rest of my life if it means that I feel physically good and not grotesquely stuffed, with my mind filled with guilt for what I cannot undo. I do know what I am missing. I am missing the addiction, the guilt, and the mental bashing that for me comes as the price for eating processed sugar.

Everyone's body is different. I have learned what works for my body and what doesn't work for it in order for me and my body to thrive.

How else do I know that sugar is an addictive substance for me, an allergen to my body? I know because I have no desire for it. Without the presence of sugar in my body, my body and mind do not crave it. When a certain amount of processed sugar is present in my body, my body and mind feel an unsatisfying need for more.

I have a very strong belief about sugar and meat, so strong, that I do not sit around and think about cheeseburgers and chocolate like I once used to.

This is what I mean by eating what you believe in. When you believe strongly in something, you are no longer swayed by the thoughts of, "What if I just ate one?"

There are cultures that eat different food groups than ours in the United States. Most people in the United States would never eat dog or horse. It is part of our cultural belief system that we just don't do that. Thus, most people in the US are not tempted to eat dog or horse.

But you have to get educated, and you have to listen to your body, you have to build that relationship.

Educate yourself on processed sugar and imitation sugars and sweeteners and their addictive qualities and see if those substances are ones that you believe are good for your body or not. I have read many articles and books that mention sugar's addictive qualities as well as sugar making weight loss more difficult. This also includes the use of sugar substitutes.

When I was in the 12-step program many years ago, one of the things they suggested eliminating from one's daily food intake was sugar and white flours because of their addictive properties. Now, for me, I can eat products from white flours and I do not feel any addictive side effects, but with sugary desserts I do. So I don't eat desserts, but I do eat white flour products, when, of course, it is something that my body wants to eat.

If like me, there are certain food groups that you cannot say no to, or can't stop eating once you start, take a look at that; acknowledge that. It's okay. There's nothing wrong with you. It's just the way your body reacts for whatever reasons it does. These types of foods I call trigger foods.

Chapter 18

Trigger Foods

For years, I kept an almost empty fridge because there wasn't much I could keep around if it were there. When I attended the 12-step program, they talked about being aware of those trigger foods and not having them in your house. I made a list of those, and the list was long. I stopped stocking my fridge and shelves with the foods that were on that list.

One of those foods for me was peanut butter. I could eat it by the spoonful and lose control, so I stopped buying peanut butter. For ten years, I did not eat peanut butter. Only in the last couple of years have I had some. But when I buy it now, I buy a single serving packet. I don't buy it every time I go to the store either. I buy it when it feels right. I am not afraid that I will lose control with peanut butter now, because I don't have that desire for more when the packet is done, but I am aware that at one time I couldn't keep it around without binging on half a jar of it. I am still respectful of what I know about my past reactions and habits with food.

There are many foods that are now back in my diet that I can eat in small portions, but I know that at one time they were trigger foods for me. I do not buy large bags of potato chips or tortilla chips, but I will have some at a party, or I will have nachos at a restaurant if that's what my body is truly asking of me. Another reason I don't buy these kinds of foods is because it is a processed food. Many brand names these days use MSG in their chips. MSG is a flavor enhancer that makes people want to eat more. Some people get migraines from eating MSG. Educate yourself. Google MSG and you will find all kinds of articles on it related to numerous diseases, inflammations, and addictions in the body.

Once you have looked at food labels and researched what is in your food, your belief system will change. You will no longer be holding the bag of potato chips saying, "Just one more."

You will look at that bag of chips and think, "Eww, gross. I am not putting that in my body!"

Now, there are definitely brands of chips that are processed without added chemicals and that are also organic. Those are what I choose to buy if I do choose to buy those foods.

I am not depriving myself of anything; instead I am aware of what works for me and what doesn't.

You probably know which foods you just can't seem to get enough of.

One of my Italian language classmates one day had mentioned that he LOVES Nutella, but he doesn't buy it. He said that if he has Nutella in the house, he will eat the whole thing in one sitting by the spoonful. Now that's a man that knows one of his trigger foods.

Take a paper and pen, identify and create your list of trigger foods. Here are some things to ask yourself as you are creating the list:

1) Do I feel guilty after I eat this food?
2) When I am eating this food, do I intend to stop eating after a certain amount, but then keep taking one more bite?
3) If the food is in the house, do I think of eating it just because it is there?

I recommend not buying trigger foods and not keeping them in the house. A recovering alcoholic doesn't keep a bottle in the house. Someone who quits smoking doesn't carry a pack of cigarettes on them. Someone who wants to stay away from foods that create an addictive reaction is better off not having the addictive foods around. Of course, it's always your choice what you choose to eat, whether it is there or not. I just found this to be a helpful tool.

There was a time when my cabinets and refrigerator were basically empty other than some nuts, vegetables, fruit, bread, and some eggs. Yes, at one time, almost everything was a trigger food for me! Pretty much if I saw it, I ate it. I had to relearn how to eat, and I had to relearn how to have food in the house. Over time, I was able to add a food or two into my house without it consuming my thoughts. Now, I can have any food, and it doesn't matter, because I choose to ask my body what it wants to eat, and I don't consider foods that go against my belief system.

A student of *The Love Your Body Class* asked me one time, "What if you have a family and you have to have different foods around that may be trigger foods for you?"

Here's my suggestion, talk to your family. Let them know what you are dealing with; ask them for their help, and as a family come up with a plan. Hopefully, they are willing to support you. Don't keep this a secret, this is one of the reasons you are facing this issue in the first place. And if you must have trigger foods in the house, by identifying what those are, and asking yourself before you eat anything, "How will I feel after I eat this?" you will probably not even want to touch those trigger foods.

As an educator, I believe strongly in the power of education. When I was a freshman in college, I had a Sociology teacher who repeatedly referred to the quote by Francis Bacon, "Knowledge is Power."

To add to this idea, knowledge is only power if you do something with it, if you are able to take action and make choices because of your knowledge. Know your trigger foods and choose not to touch them. You are not depriving yourself of anything special; you are keeping a binge at bay and the guilt away.

Chapter 19

Being Present with Your Food

In order to continue living, surviving, and thriving, people must eat. Everyone knows that. That is why our bodies give us the signal of hunger. In our fast-paced society and busy lives, so many people are eating on the run, popping a TV dinner in the microwave and eating it while they are getting ready, or stopping at a popular fast food drive-thru on their way from work to an appointment or to some other committed activity. Some people eat at the fridge with the intention of just one bite, which then leads to one more bite, and then one more bite, until it's too late and they feel they have blown it again. Others eat what they are "supposed" to be eating based on the latest diet trend.

Eating is a gift. Food is a gift for our bodies. Our bodies are not who we are, we are the spirit within our bodies. Your spirit wants to connect with your body in the pleasure of eating the food that gives it nourishment and life force. If you are constantly eating on the run, eating at the counter or the fridge, or following some diet that tells you what to eat and yet you are not happy about what you are eating, then you are not giving your spirit the time to connect with your body and you are not honoring your body.

When you make the time to sit and eat and be with the food you eat, you will find a peaceful enjoyment that comes out of it, completely opposite from devouring something that you think is bad for you but tastes good and wanting more even though you are full. While your body is saying it's full, your spirit is saying it's still empty. This is one of the reasons people overeat. This is one of the reasons they cannot stop even though they are sick to their stomach with fullness.

Before every meal, I have made it a conscious habit to be aware of the food I am eating. First of all, I always ask my body what it would like to eat. Remember, we are spirits in our bodies, we are not our bodies. We have a relationship with our bodies.

When you are in a relationship with a man or a woman and you plan to go out for dinner, do you drag them to any restaurant that you feel like, or do you ask them, "What would you like to eat?"

"What are you in the mood for?"

That is a way of acknowledging and honoring your partner, and when you honor your partner, aren't they happy with you? Aren't they happy with you for considering their thoughts, feelings, needs, wants, and desires? Of course, they are. When you honor your partner, does your relationship grow and strengthen? Of course, it does. It's the same with your body. If you are not honoring your body, you are probably disconnected from it. When we are in relationships where we become disconnected, what happens? They stop working well.

Try this before your next meal, ask, "Body, what would you like to eat?" and listen.

Before eating breakfast in the morning, ask yourself, "Body, what would you like to eat?"

You may surprise yourself with what you feel or hear back from your body. It may not be part of your regular breakfast routine. It may be something totally different.

For years, I had an egg with whole wheat toast for breakfast. I felt it was safe. It was 100 calories for a slice of bread and 70 calories for the egg, while keeping me full until lunch time. Now that I ask my body what it wants to eat, I rarely eat the same thing two mornings in a row. I used to have all of these rules like: *I must eat breakfast; people who eat breakfast have a higher metabolism. I must have 2 glasses of water first thing in the morning to speed up my metabolism.*

Now, I just ask my body what it wants.

In fact, just this morning I woke up and asked my body what it wanted and then prepared myself a green salad with Italian scallions, yellow bell peppers, and cherry tomatoes. I sprinkled some sea salt on it and added some organic olive oil. I sat down at my kitchen table, looked at my breakfast, and thanked God for the food that I had before me.

A client of mine said that for years she forced herself to eat breakfast because she had heard that eating breakfast speeds up the metabolism. When she started asking her body if it was truly hungry, she found that her body did not like eating breakfast. We all have different bodies and they have different needs and requirements, so ask your body what it needs and what it requires.

Before eating I always, always, always give thanks. Most often I say the same prayer, but always I give thanks. I usually say, "Dear God, thank you for this food. Please make it good for my body, healthy for my body, and just what my body needs."

Sometimes, I will also ask for Him to make the food healing for my body.

Before I eat, I always look at my food. Gratitude is an important part of eating, because you are gifting your body, and in return gifting the relationship that you have with your body. Gratitude aids you in being present with your food and tasting your food.

Taking your time to eat and being "with" your food can be challenging at first if this is not your habit. But give yourself grace. The more you practice, the more second nature it will become for you to eat slowly and enjoy your food and really taste every bite, tasting the textures and the flavors.

Usually, I am the last one at the table still eating. One time a guy that I was dating said, "I noticed that you don't talk and eat at the same time, you do one or the other."

He said this as he was noticing that he was always finished long before I was. This is true, but I hadn't noticed that I do one or the other. I do know that I trained myself to taste my food, to enjoy it, and to savor every bite that I put in my mouth. I do not like to talk while I have food in my mouth.

When I started slowing down my eating and truly tasting the textures, the juices, and the flavors, I started thinking about food less.

I stopped wondering when my next meal was. I stopped thinking about how I shouldn't want to eat because I'm not hungry now, but I want to anyway. The craziness slowed down for me because I was being present with what I was eating. I was cultivating and nurturing the relationship I have with my body, as well as food. At the time, I wasn't aware that I had a relationship with my body at all. I just knew that thinking in this way seemed to help me with my food obsession cravings.

When I first became aware of slowing down how quickly I ate and focusing on tasting my food, I had to be really conscious of this act. At the time, it was good for me that I was single and ate most of my dinners by myself, because then I could really focus on what I was eating and not a conversation. Another thing I began to practice, when I was eating by myself, was eating as if someone else was there with me.

Enjoy every bite that goes into your mouth, it is a gift to feed our body good healthy food so that our system can function at its best.

Being Present with the Food You Eat

- Before eating, ask yourself, "Am I truly hungry? How will I feel after I eat this? Will I feel guilty from any of the food that I am choosing?"
- Only put on your plate what your body wants at this meal. Ask, "Body, how much of this food do you require?"
- Sit down to eat your snack, your meal, or anything that you are going to eat.
- Bless your food, thank God, and thank the food.
- Taste each bite.
- Don't put another bite into your mouth until you are fully finished with the bite before it.
- Eat slowly, very slowly, as slow as you can.
- Once you are finished with the meal, do not get up for a second helping; let your body digest the amount of food it said it required.
- When you are finished with your meal, thank God, and thank the food.

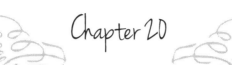

Chapter 20

An Example of Listening to My Body

Once, I had a really strong cold. I went to the grocery store and spent $40 on a bunch of organic vegetables so as to create a "healthy" soup. My friend said to me, "The good thing about being sick is that you eat all of the things you should be eating."

Ha, interesting point of view for her to say that. Interesting that I thought I should make this soup and eat it in the first place. When the soup was finished cooking and I began eating it, I thought how boring this soup was. It just wasn't satisfying at all. Then I realized that I hadn't even asked my body what it wanted to eat. I went into my old points of view and beliefs that when one is sick, one should eat soup.

I asked my body, "If you could eat anything right now, what would it be?"

It said, "Pizza."

I said, "Pizza? But I won't even be able to taste it right now."

I made the pizza anyway. If it turned out that I wasn't interested in it when it was ready, I could just put it in a plastic baggie and throw it back in the fridge for another day. I took the frozen Margherita pizza out of the freezer and placed some jalapenos over it. Then I put it in the oven to bake for 10 minutes. I got my plate ready with Caesar dressing for dipping, and when the pizza was golden, I took it out to cool off. I cut my little pizza into eight little slices, put them on my plate and headed back to my bed where I'd been hibernating with the cold I'd had. Lo and behold I could taste the pizza! It was delicious! It was what my body wanted, just like it had said, and I was truly satisfied afterwards.

It was just a reminder to me that it is so much easier to just ask my body what it wants, and then to honor that.

Chapter 21

There is No Waste

I know many people who finish everything on their plate because they don't want to waste any food. I used to be one of these people, or I would eat the last few chips because I thought it was silly to put only a few back in the cupboard or to throw them away.

Well, there are different ways that you can look at this, and different perspectives that you can choose to take. I say "choose" because whatever you choose to believe is *your* truth. It is not truth for everyone. At one time my truth was that leaving any extra food was a waste, but now my truth has changed.

My perspective on this is that there is no waste, because it's all waste! The food either goes in your mouth, through your digestive system, and it exits your body as waste, or you can choose to throw it away and it will decompose in the landfill and it also becomes waste. Either way the food becomes waste from your body or waste into the garbage can after it decomposes. But, remember this, your body is not a trash can!

When your body has told you that it has had enough to eat, you can choose to continue eating so that you don't "waste" any food and, thus, in return hurt your body and your relationship with it by not listening, or you can choose to listen to your body and honor it by not finishing the food. Either way, in the end, it all decomposes and becomes waste. Your choice.

I have heard from people, "But there are children starving in Africa!!!"

We've all heard that line, right? My response to that is, "Can you affect those starving children in Africa right now with the food that is in front of you?"

The answer is no, you can't. What should concern you is that you have been gifted with the ability to take care of you in this moment and there is no reason to feel guilty for this.

Many people grew up in families where their parents said, "You must finish your plate if you want dessert," or "You must eat everything on your plate. Don't waste any food."

Our beliefs about food and the stories that play out in our head are usually stories that we have picked up from our caregivers and the media.

Pay attention to your thoughts about wasting food and when they occur. Ask yourself if these thoughts are really true or are a belief you picked up on, and consider whether following that belief will hurt you or honor you? Will it hurt your body or will it be kind to your body?

There really is no waste, because in the end, it all decomposes, so it's all waste.

Chapter 22

Get Honest with Yourself

Get straight with yourself about what you want. Do you truly want to be free from the craziness of yo-yo dieting and being abusive to your body or do you still want that lifestyle? Because it is a lifestyle. I have met people who have told me they don't want to make any changes; they just want to lose weight or be skinny. My question to them always is, "If you keep doing what you have been doing, won't you continue to get more of what you have been getting?"

No one ever said changing your lifestyle was effortless. It takes work and dedication and it is not always comfortable, but you live through it one day at a time, and you look at the blessings and gifts that you have received from creating change.

Is your current lifestyle comfortable? If you are here reading this book, looking for answers, or looking to make a change in your life, then perhaps it's not. Over time, your new lifestyle will flow with more ease, and one day you will notice that your new lifestyle has become effortless and a part of you.

I'm not offering you a diet or a promise of weight loss. I'm offering you tools and ideas that you can use to create a new lifestyle for yourself, full of freedom from diet addiction and body obsession, which then results in a body that you love. Weight loss is often a natural occurring result of honoring your body. Your body stabilizes to the place and weight that is healthy for it.

Sometimes, I encounter people who have an excuse for every tool I offer them. They do not want to put the effort in that it takes to create change and they are afraid of "losing control" of their weight. They were never in control of their weight in the first place. The only control they have is how they choose to treat their body, with love and kindness or with hate and unkindness. Then their body responds to that which they give their body.

One woman I had a conversation with said, "I don't have an issue with my weight, I just want to be thin and eat whatever I want."

I asked her, "Why are you seeing a nutritionist? Why are you weighing yourself on the scale? And why have you sought out a body relationship session with me? Stop bullshitting yourself! If you had no issue and didn't want some kind of change to occur, we would not be talking right now."

Be really honest with yourself. Do you want to make this change and commitment in your life? If you are ready, fantastic! You will be blessed with bliss from the creations that come from your choices. Give yourself grace and patience as you make these changes. There may be times when you truly forget to ask your body what it wants to eat, or you make a choice that does result in guilt. Remember that every moment is a new moment and in each moment you have the power to choose.

Please understand that I know it can be scary to let go of control and to trust your body, but your body truly will change its form into a form that you will love when you honor it and love it. It can't hurt to go for it, especially if what you have been doing, has not been working.

So, be true to yourself. Are you in this half way or the whole way? If you are here to "try" this out for a couple of days, it's not enough. That's the same thinking of "trying" a diet out for a few days and then falling off the wagon and eating everything in sight until you get on your next diet. Make a commitment to yourself to do this, to ask your body questions, to show your body gratitude, to be kind to your body and to honor it, and see what miraculous changes occur in your spirit, your body, and your soul. You have probably spent many years programming your mind and body to think the way it does. It takes 21 days to break a habit. Start reprogramming the way you think and react about your body, and see how incredible life can be when you treat yourself with love and respect.

I know in this chapter I am serious, straightforward, and maybe even a little harsh, but making excuses to not get something done, never accomplished anything. Do you care about yourself enough to give yourself the love, effort, and time to create a happy, healthy relationship with your body???

If you choose to continue your same lifestyle, ask yourself, "Why am I continuing to do something I claim makes me unhappy?" and then don't judge your answer, just ask.

Chapter 23

Moving Your Body

Most people call it exercise or working out, but I like to call it moving your body. Personally, I "worked out" for many years and hated it half of the time. That term to me means being in a gym or making my body do something that it doesn't feel like doing.

There are many people out there who get their body moving without feeling like it is something they have to do. They participate in a sport that they love such as soccer, tennis, rowing, cycling, etc... These people are fortunate that they have found a way to move their body that is honoring to them.

Moving your body is important for your overall health. It is good for your cardiovascular system. It can prevent and manage all kinds of health issues and concerns. It releases certain chemicals in your brain that make you feel happier. It can boost your self-esteem because you feel better about your body when you move it. It increases your connection to your body. It increases your energy. It also keeps your muscles strong.

It is an incredible energy booster. When I taught elementary school in Westminster, Colorado, I would be so tired after lunch that I felt like I could barely move. Some days getting through a math lesson was excruciatingly painful. When I started incorporating walks into my 40-minute lunch period, my whole afternoon changed. It was like a miracle! I was no longer tired after lunch. Instead, I was refreshed and ready to teach math. On the days where I would skip the walk because I had too much to do and thought I needed to work through my lunch, I found that I was really sluggish on those afternoons. Eventually, I made it a habit to go for a walk every single day at lunch. It was something my body needed and craved. It was also good for my spirit as it gave me time to be with nature, to be with me, and to be with God.

When you move your body in a way that is honoring to your body, it nurtures your relationship with your body and it nurtures your spirit. Movement connects us to our body, making us consciously aware of feeling our spirit in our body and feeling the sensations that occur in our body from the movement. Movement also brings peace to our spirit because it is grounding.

Moving is important to keep your body strong. Have you ever seen an elderly person that moves really slowly? It is possible this person stopped moving their body consistently at some point. I have a firm belief that if you continue to move your body every day or at least almost every day, then you will always be able to move. Your body will not slow down because of old age. My grandfather, who lived into his 90's, continued to walk, take stairs, and play tennis until the end of his life. His body was like that of a 20-year-old, but he rarely went a day without moving.

Ask your body how you can honor it through movement. If it is hitting up the gym, then by all means hit up the gym, lift weights, climb on the elliptical or the treadmill, but if that is not what honors your body, then choose for it what does. Your body knows what kind of movement it would like to make. Movement is so much more fun and enjoyable when it is aligned with what your body and spirit desire. When your motivation to move is because your body wants it and not because you are thinking you need to work out to lose weight, moving your body comes with ease. What results is a beautiful and strong body.

I rarely go to the gym, but every once in a while I get an itch to lift weights. On most occasions for me, the gym is not honoring to my body. Usually, I go for a walk, take lots of stairs, and do jumping jacks, lunges, pushups, and crunches. My body likes that. It feels good when it moves in these ways, and I never have to drag myself to do any of these movements. My body and my spirit prefer to be outside when I move.

Sometimes I move my body for a couple of hours at a time and sometimes for 15 minutes. It just depends, but I don't force my body into anything. So, whereas it used to be a drag to have to work out every day, now I move my body every day of the week, unless when I ask it, it doesn't want to move. It usually does want to move in some form though every day.

You may or may not find working out fun. Just listen to the term... working... out. It's work! I know many people, who move their bodies every day, but it's not by force, it is something they want to do. It's usually a sport such as biking or soccer, and they do it because they love to be outdoors, enjoy nature, and they love the way it feels to move their body in that way.

Moving your body gives your body the opportunity to take on a toned form, but if your motivation is for looks alone, it can be a real drag. If your motivation is because you are choosing a movement your body loves and a movement your spirit enjoys making, then it will be something you want to get out there and do often. For instance, I love tennis! My body loves the way it feels to stroke the ball with my racket or to sprint up to the net and send the ball into the back of my opponent's court. I love the competition of a one on one game! This is movement that my body loves and my spirit loves, and my body reaps all of the health benefits when I get out there to play a match.

Ask your body:

"Body, what types of movements are good for you?"

"Body, what kinds of movement would you like to make?"

"Body, would you like to move today, and if so, what would you like to do to move?"

You can ask your body however you want, but just ask. If your body gives you an answer that you don't believe is good for weight loss, follow what your body desires, because if you are working out for weight loss then you are still in the dieting cycle of abuse. You are forcing your body to do something that it may not want to do. Trust that your body knows what it needs.

You can ask, "Body what kind of movement would you like to do today that will be nourishing to you?"

You know how some people do certain workouts that create injuries in their body? Those injuries or pains are their body's way of letting them know that it doesn't like what is being done. If exercise is done for health, and you are injuring your body, then how is that affecting your health?

When I was in college, I used to run almost every day. I developed knee pain in my left knee, but I kept running on it because I believed that I had to run in order to lose weight. I finally listened to it when I really couldn't run on it anymore. Luckily, I did not have to have surgery like many other people I know.

If we don't listen to the messages that our body is giving us, they will get loud enough that one day you have to listen or pay major consequences. For me, that would have been having knee surgery. I was just lucky the pain became too intense for me even to walk on it and I had to make a change. I was fortunate I finally listened.

I used to go religiously to the gym for cardio and to lift weights. In the past, I worked out for weight and for my health. Even after my obsession with food was gone, I still went to the gym for my health and for body strength. Most of my adult life, I have had a personal trainer that I have met with at least once a week, because I have never had the personal motivation to go to the gym. I have never loved it at all.

My last trainer and dear friend, would have to listen to me complain for the entire hour, throughout our session, about all of the exercises he was having me do.

Once he asked me point blank, "Why are you paying me to do this if you hate it so much?"

"I am paying you because I wouldn't do it otherwise. I have to be accountable to someone," I told him.

I had this belief that I could only move my body, stay healthy, and get in shape by lifting weights and doing intense cardio. Now, I have a different perspective. Now, I ask my body what kind of movement it would like to do, just as I ask my body what it wants to eat.

What if you chose to move your body because it was honoring your body and your relationship with your body?

What if you chose to move your body because it made you feel incredibly alive?

What kinds of movement make your body happy and healthy?

What kind of movement is available to you out there that you have never even considered before that could add so much joy and happiness to your body and spirit?

Would you be willing to let go of exercise being a must-do and start asking your body how it would like to move?

Chapter 24

Choice

One day, it occurred to me that the only day I had to worry about what I put in my mouth was today. The only meal I had to think about what to eat was the meal I was about to have now. I could not change what I had already eaten and I could not in this moment change my body. I realized I could only affect change by the choices I made in this current moment.

I reached a point where I could not stand the guilt I was constantly enduring for what I had eaten two days ago, last night, or for what I had just put in my mouth. The guilt was like a constant siren in my head that was so loud I couldn't escape it.

Then, if I had chosen to throw up the food I had eaten or eaten foods that I was afraid would make me fat, I would feel guilty once again for choosing to stick my head in the toilet, but the guilt didn't end there. The next day, I had to endure the icky sensation of a sore throat scraped by my own fingers. In my desperation to be thin, I was happy that I could get rid of food from my body. I was happy I could make myself throw up. I just didn't like the guilt.

The first time I was successful at purging food from my body, I was living in San Diego and I was 23 years old. I had tried many times before to make myself throw up and I was never successful. I had always been so frustrated about it.

One night I was in Old Town with some friends, and we had just had Mexican food for dinner. Sitting at the dinner table and feeling overridden with guilt for eating too much, I headed to the bathroom to try and alleviate my once again disgustingly full stomach, and voila, this time I succeeded. I remember being so happy and proud of myself that this time I was able to throw up my food. I will never forget walking out of that bathroom on a warm spring night, feeling the wetness of my eyes that comes with vomiting, and smiling all the way back to the table. I had succeeded. Yes, I had succeeded in beginning a new habit and pattern.

The days with my head in the toilet lasted for a solid three years and I never felt like I was that bad, because I didn't do it every day. In fact, I justified that it was okay because I only threw up 3-4 times per week, and I wasn't like other people who did it every time they ate.

But I did keep it a secret from the people in my life. If I was with family or friends and I chose to throw up my food, I usually went through a hurried routine in the bathroom so that they wouldn't notice. I would quickly fix my makeup, because my eyes would tear up and my black eyeliner would run down along the sides of my face. Then I would have to pop a piece of gum and chew it quickly, and put a cold compress of water and a paper towel under my eyes. I didn't want any questions and I felt that I didn't need any lectures.

When I was 26 years old, my father died, and along with his death I stopped throwing my food up for the most part. After he died, nothing seemed to matter anymore, and I couldn't stomach putting anything in my mouth. I had no appetite and thus nothing to feel guilty about for eating. When my father died, I saw things differently and I thought it was so silly what I was doing.

I saw everything differently in my life. Everything that was once big and important in my life became small and meaningless. Caring so much about my weight became silly to me, it became non-important.

It wasn't like I was miraculously "normal," but my perception changed about what was important and what wasn't. In the years after I stopped purging on a regular basis, I threw up maybe a handful of times, but that was largely the end of my head in the toilet.

I also came to the conclusion that if I was going to choose to eat something, then I was going to keep it down. If I chose to put it in my body, I was going to choose not to stick my fingers down my throat and throw it up. I had enough of throwing up, and I knew my father would be proud of me for this choice. I also knew that I was proud of myself when I chose not to purge my food.

One day I realized that no matter how much I tried to control the future of my weight today, my weight today was what it was. I could not change that now. I could only make choices now that could affect change. I realized that in the end, I am not in control of any of it, and this is where my weight obsession had held its power over me. I wanted the control, and I had the belief that I had it, and yet I never seemed to be at the weight I wanted to be, never! It wouldn't matter if I dropped 5 pounds, because then I would think I would only be happy if I dropped 5 more, and if I dropped 5 more, I would only be happy if I lost 2 more pounds. It occurred to me that I would never, ever, ever, in a million years be happy with my body, and so I chose to work on the guilt and not the weight.

So for each meal I started asking myself, "What can I eat that will not give me guilt?"

"What can I eat that I will feel okay about myself after I eat it?"

I started eating based on how I would feel emotionally and physically after each meal and each thing I put in my mouth. I had reached a point where I hated, and I mean loathed, feeling too full or any kind of fullness at all. I had reached a point where I hated the feeling of guilt more than I wanted to be in control of my weight, and what resulted were those questions. When you want one thing more than the other thing, change can happen with much more ease.

If you are someone who tends to feel guilty after you have eaten or even while you are eating, before you make your dinner or order your dinner, ask yourself, "What can I eat that will not give me guilt?"

Ask your body, "Body what would you like to eat?"

If you ask both of these questions together, you will be intuitively directed to choose a meal that leaves you satisfied and guilt-free.

In the beginning stages of discovering freedom from food and weight obsession, I found that if I wanted to make a choice that I knew I would feel guilty about making, I would tell myself that I could have that food tomorrow if I still wanted it, and I meant it. If I was still really craving those nachos or cheeseburger or French fries or cheesecake or whatever it was, I could have it tomorrow.

There were times when I still wanted those foods the next day and I asked myself if I would feel guilty and the answer was no. Then I ate them, and there was no guilt attached to eating them.

I applied this same method of thinking to when I had quit smoking and really wanted to have a cigarette, even though I knew that if I did I would feel horrible and the guilt would tear me up. There have been times when I had been triggered to smoke and I would have to tell myself that for today I had made the choice not to smoke, and if I still felt this incredible desire tomorrow, then by all means, I had my own permission to make that choice tomorrow.

Always, I was so grateful that I gave myself the choice. Choice is freedom. I don't know about you, but if you tell me that I can't have something, then that's probably the first thing that I want to have, but if you give me a choice, then I can react calmly to the situation and make a decision I will feel good about. Give yourself choice. We all want what we can't have, and when you give yourself choice, mean it.

As human beings, we thrive on choice, no matter what the substance or situation is, but if our choice is taken away from us, we will want what we can't have.

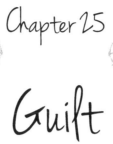

Chapter 25

Guilt

Ahhhh, guilt! If there is one feeling in this world I run from and avoid at all costs, it is guilt. Guilt creates an anxiety in me that I find nearly unbearable. It makes me feel uneasy, unintelligent, and uncomfortable in my own skin. It makes me want to run and hide, although there is nowhere for me to run to. I cannot escape my head. That's where the guilt lives, in my head. I have had to learn how *to be* with thoughts that create feelings of unease within me.

Guilt is a feeling created in response to doing something wrong or in response to something that you believe is wrong. I used to experience guilt when I would eat certain foods or eat too much of any type of food. Was it wrong for me to eat half a cheeseburger with French fries and ranch dressing? In reality there is nothing right or wrong about that, it's all based on one's point of view and perception about that meal. However, I have learned that if I experience guilt in regard to any situation, I am not being true to myself on some level.

It was very rare that I could eat a cheeseburger and fries without feeling guilty about it, and it was my favorite meal. It was part of my belief system that cheeseburgers and fries put together would make me fat and that they are unhealthy. On top of all of that, eating that meal would always leave me feeling extra full and heavy.

For me, the feeling of full and heavy is not comfortable. If I eat to the point of being too full, then I am not honoring my body. My body does not like to feel full or stuffed. It just doesn't. My body does not like the feeling of fullness. It doesn't feel free. It feels tired, restricted, and distracted by the pressure of feeling full.

I discovered that when I eat foods that create guilt within me, I am not being true to myself and I am not honoring my relationship with my body.

It helps to identify those foods that you feel guilty about after you have eaten them. Foods that make you feel guilty after you eat them are different than trigger foods. A trigger food will definitely leave you feeling guilty, but a trigger food is when you start eating something and you feel that you cannot stop eating more of that particular food and it leads to a binge.

A food that creates guilt is a food that you have created a particular belief around. For instance, I used to believe that fried foods would make me fat, and so if I ate anything fried, I would feel guilty afterwards. I believed that nachos would make me fat, so if I ate nachos, I would feel guilty after. I believed that desserts would make me fat, and so every time I ate dessert, I would feel guilty.

Here is why I highly suggest identifying what foods make you feel guilty and then not eating those, because if you don't feel guilty, you break the cycle of abuse on your body.

I had a client that once said to me, "Well if I can't eat these foods from my guilty list, I'm afraid I am going to feel deprived."

My response to her was, "The only thing you are depriving yourself of is guilt. You always have the choice to eat anything you want, but why would you choose to eat something that you know is going to leave you feeling guilty?"

In a relationship between a man and a woman, when one person cheats on the other, that person usually feels guilty. This guilt is in response to them not honoring their current relationship. The person who has cheated, usually feels they have betrayed themselves and the person they love, and risked the trust in their relationship.

When comparing relationships with people, to eating and food, we can compare this situation to the term, "I cheated on my diet."

However, the "diet" is what is coming between you and your relationship with your body. You're not cheating on your diet. You're cheating on you. You're cheating on your body with the diet. Instead of letting your body do its part in the relationship by taking care of how it processes food, you turn to something else, such as a diet.

The word *diet* really means what you eat on a regular basis, but a "diet" that you do for a short period of time to obtain results in the short term (even though you think it's for the long term), is cheating on your relationship with your body.

Many years ago, I began asking myself when looking at a menu in a restaurant, "Will this make me feel guilty while I am eating it, immediately after I am eating it, the next day or even a few days later?"

If the answer was yes, I had a choice to make.

That's all it was and still is: a choice.

I didn't and don't have to make this choice for the rest of my meals for the rest of my life. I only have to make this choice for the current meal. For this is the only meal that is present right now and that I have the present choice in.

Guilt for me is now a rarity. If I do eat too much, which happens on a rare occasion, I am only a little too full and not a lot. I also know that it is one meal and I can choose again for my next meal. I do not feel the need to continue to beat myself up for it and feel guilty. I deserve grace, as do you.

If you tend to feel guilty after you eat, ask yourself beforehand, "Will I feel guilty after I eat this?" Then you can choose if you would still like to eat what will make you feel guilty or you can choose to not eat it. By asking this question before choosing to eat something, you bring awareness to yourself about what you are going to do. Awareness changes everything.

If what you choose to eat results in guilt, why would you choose to eat it?

For everything you are going to choose to eat or drink, before making that choice, ask yourself, "Will this make me feel guilty or not guilty?"

"How will I feel after I eat this?"

To say you have no control over what you put in your mouth is not true, and to say that you can't help yourself, is also not true as well. It may not be easy, it may be hard and uncomfortable at first, but it's always a choice. *You have wired your brain to think in a certain way and you have created a certain way of choosing.*

Always question your body and question your choices before you make them. This creates awareness and awareness changes everything!

If you are going to choose to eat something that makes you feel guilty after you eat it, then before you eat it, say out loud, "I am choosing to eat this, even though I will feel guilty after I eat it."

By bringing this awareness to yourself about what you are about to do, and the consequences of it, your desire to do this harm to yourself will decrease and you may find the urge to eat what you were thinking about eating in the first place, dissipates or goes away. Your brain will go, *How silly, I am choosing to eat something that's going to make me feel like shit!*

You can ask yourself, "Am I truly hungry right now?"

If you are, and what you are choosing to eat doesn't create guilt, then great, eat it, it's good for your body. But if you're not hungry and you're going to choose to eat something then say out loud, "I'm not hungry and I am going to eat this."

I have never eaten anything after I have made myself aware in this way. It's always stopped me in my tracks and made the mental desire to eat go away. And if you feel guilty after eating most foods, then make a list of what you eat that doesn't create guilt and choose from there. You may have a short list, but it is a place to start with eliminating guilt and rewiring your brain to choose what makes you feel at peace instead of guilty. Guilt is a huge contributor in the habitual cycle of dieting. You have to break and dismantle the cycle.

If you take guilt out of the equation, your whole life will change in regards to how you look at food, your weight, and your body. Guilt is the number one contributor to you not feeling good about you.

Chapter 26

Throw it Out-Your Scale

One of the best pieces of advice I was given years ago, while I was an outpatient at a clinic in San Diego, was to throw my scale out. Of course, when my counselor there suggested that I do this, I thought she was crazy! What ran through my head went something like this (with a little added dramatics for humor):

Throw my scale out? I can't live without my scale! My scale and I are like best friends! We wake up in the morning together and we have a weigh in. My scale tells me how my day is going to be, and all about my self-worth. I won't know who I am without my scale!

My scale and I meet as soon as I get home from work because I need to be told if I am okay or if I am a fat piece of shit. This way I can either beat myself up for how disgusting I am or obsess about how to keep my weight where it is or if I need to lose just a little more.

Before getting on the scale, I most definitely undress because I don't want any extra weight that is not truly mine to show up. I most definitely take off my underwear, my bra, my earrings, my bracelets, and anything else that could possibly tip the scale by an ounce. Then I hold my breath before peeking at the numbers... up two pounds from this morning. That's okay. I have learned that during the day I am always two pounds heavier than in the evening. If it were 3 pounds, well, then I would definitely have to give myself a beating and figure out how did I put on that extra pound today? Am I bloated, getting my period? What did I eat last night? Hmmm, maybe it was the kidney beans in the salad, they are carbohydrates...

Next, I put my clothes back on and put myself back together, so that I can get on with the evening, and depending on the day or should I say the number on the scale, I may just turn right back around and strip down to my birthday suit just to make sure that the number wasn't off a half of a pound.

Before going to bed, my best friend and I always get together at least one more time. This way I will know when I am trying to go to sleep if I should be counting up in my head the calories I had for the day, even though that's already been done and written down, or if I should plan out all of my meals in my head for tomorrow.

Throw out my scale? Why in the world would I want to throw out the gauge of my day and my self-esteem? Who would I be without my scale? How will I know what I should think about in regards to my weight and what I can and cannot eat that day? Throw out my scale??? That's crazy!

Well, I wanted to get better. I was tired of obsessing about my weight. I was tired of having conversations with friends and not being present because I was adding up calories in my head while talking to them. I was tired of being addicted to thinking about my weight. I was tired of starving. I was tired of overeating. I was tired of throwing up. I was tired of taking laxatives. I was tired of hating my body. I was tired of hating myself. I was tired of being a slave to the thoughts that ran around in my brain. I was willing to try anything. So after acknowledging my fears about not having a scale anymore, I agreed to let mine go.

It wasn't like I just went home and threw it out. No, I had to look at it for a while. I had to weigh myself one more time. I had to talk to it and tell it why I was letting it go. How "they" say it's not healthy for me to own a scale. How I loved it, but had to let it go. How what we had was an abusive relationship, and the only way to end the cycle of abuse, was to end the relationship.

It was an early evening in San Diego and the sun was still blazing. I held my white digital scale in my arms and walked it to the big green dumpster that sat twenty yards from the entrance of my apartment. I just stood there. I didn't want to part with my friend. For the past 11 years or so, there wasn't a day that went by that I didn't check in. It was like breaking up with a guy that I was crazy about, but that I knew was not good for me. I was very afraid to let it go. But I did; one, two, three. I counted to three and then tossed it into the dumpster.

I was okay for the moment, but I felt very anxious and nervous about not having my scale. How was I going to manage my weight and not let my weight get out of control? I guess like any habit you kick, sometimes you just have to go cold turkey.

Parting with my friend was hard. There were days when I missed her terribly and just wanted to know what I weighed, but most days I was okay. I think because I was working with a treatment center and this was something I wanted, to be free of this weight obsession. I was willing to make some changes.

I won't lie; I had other ways of measuring myself. One of these ways was to take my hand and wrap it around the bicep part of my arm, and just by feel I could tell where I was. Although it didn't give me a number, it gave me an idea that my body wasn't growing.

I also had to throw out my measuring tape. I had only been using that for about 6 months. The tape measure certainly never made me feel good; I couldn't tell if I was placing the tape in the right area or if it was off a millimeter or two, so I threw that away too.

I haven't weighed myself purposely in 7 years. I haven't owned a scale in about 13 years. What I did find, was that giving up the scale freed me from a large fraction of the obsession. It was one piece of the puzzle that kept my self-worth tied to a number. It was one large part of the cycle of self-abuse in my obsession with my weight. When I removed one of the largest objects of my obsession, a lot of the pressure seemed to fall away. The worry in my head about my weight became quieter, and did not seem to rule every single second of my day or every thought that entered my mind.

After a few years of living without weighing in, I found myself returning to the scale. In 2005, I moved from San Diego to Denver to start a new teaching position. I was happy with my weight. I was still concerned and watched what I ate, but for the most part, I had reached a place where I didn't feel crazy.

I was so busy my first year of teaching that I would literally forget to eat lunch or dinner. I would start eating a meal, and then get side tracked on a school project and forget that I was even eating in the first place. People were telling me I looked really skinny. I felt really good about that and I would go downstairs to the gym in my apartment complex and work out every morning before school started, because I wanted to maintain my skinniness.

There was a scale in the gym and I was feeling pretty confident that I did not have an issue with food or my weight anymore, so one morning I decided to weigh myself. The scale read 113 pounds. *Okay*, I thought, *that's great*, and I continued to think about how great that was. As I thought about how great it was that I weighed 113 pounds, I innocently began counting my calories, not so that I could lose weight, but so that I could maintain it. Then I began weighing myself at the gym more often, until sometimes what motivated me to get to the gym was the fact that I could jump on the scale there.

I am not sure that I recognized anything changing within me or any of my old patterns returning, until one day I was sitting at my computer at school around 9am and thinking about how I couldn't wait for lunch to come so that I could eat. It wasn't because I was hungry, I just wanted to eat.

I decided to have just one piece of chocolate from the bag that I had bought for my students for our Halloween party, and then I had another, and then another. I don't remember how many pieces I ate, but it scared me because I couldn't stop, and that was an all too familiar feeling. I vowed I would not do that again. However, what I didn't realize was that I was already in the cycle of abusing my body. I was feeling guilty and vowed I would not overeat ever again!

Well, the cycle continued from there. Often when elementary students celebrate their birthdays at school, they bring around treats like doughnuts and cookies and offer them to the teachers. I would take one to be polite with the intention to save it and throw it away later. There were days where I would end up with a few treats sitting on my desk with the intention of tossing them. One afternoon, just a few days after the chocolate incident, I was hungry and I ate one of the treats that were sitting on my desk. It was a cookie, and then I had the doughnut, and then I ate the other cookie, and then I felt really guilty! I vowed I would not eat treats that kids bring me, ever again!

On any given day a teacher can walk into the teacher's lounge and expect to find snacks left over from professional development the day before, half a cake from a teacher's birthday, doughnuts or cookies from a parent/child event from the morning, or a spread of leftover food from some other school event. I found that I was beginning to help myself to half a doughnut, and then the other half, and then a third of a doughnut, and then the rest of that one too. Of course, I did this when no one was looking, when the teacher's lounge was empty. Sometimes, I would make multiple trips back and forth from my outside mobile classroom to the teacher's lounge inside the school building for thirds of a doughnut, or just one more cookie. I was always left with guilt and worry that I was going to gain weight.

I realized I was spiraling out of control again, so I took myself to a 12-step meeting for people who have food and weight issues. I knew I was in trouble, and I needed help. I began working the steps again as I had just a few years before.

I also couldn't believe that every time I stepped on the scale at the gym, the number seemed to be just a little higher than the day before. I hated myself again. My jeans had become excruciatingly tight. I would look in the mirror and see a muffin top hanging over the sides of my jeans and pants. My arms were bulging; my face looked swollen, and I had a double chin in pictures. In a matter of a couple of months, I had eaten my way from 113 pounds to 134 pounds. It all started because I began focusing on my weight again.

I worked the steps. I followed the advice to eat 3 meals a day and nothing in-between. Sometimes this was extremely uncomfortable, but most of the time it wasn't. I didn't go back for seconds either. I knew my parameters. However, I still wasn't happy with going from a size 3 to a size 9. And no matter how hard I tried, I couldn't seem to drop the weight.

Then, in an attempt to get control of my weight, I joined a real gym, and invested in a personal trainer who I met with 3 times a week. Someone that I would be accountable to and someone who would root for me, and he did. Every session he looked at my food log. He even made me write down when I put a stick of gum in my mouth that was 5 calories! I went to the gym every single day for an hour of cardio and an hour of weight training. Yes, I was working out 2 hours a day, every single day, not because my trainer told me I had to, but because I wanted to drop the weight as quickly as possible.

I was on a diet of 1300 calories for the day. Often I was hungry, but I was determined to drop the weight, and at the time, restriction was the only way I knew how.

In the end, I lost the weight, and I had found some joy, but I was still counting calories. I was still afraid to gain it back, and so one day I told my trainer that when he weighed me in every week, that I didn't want to know the number anymore. I told him I was still committed to working out and writing my food down, but I couldn't know the number. I told him, "Knowing the number on the scale makes me crazy, no matter if it's 'good' or 'bad.'"

He said, "Okay."

I had realized that the reason I had gained weight in the first place, was because I had started weighing myself again and knowing my number created the desire to want to maintain that number, which led to me working out specifically for my weight and then depriving myself of food that I thought I shouldn't have, which then led to binges on those foods and me carrying around a tremendous load of guilt and shame. I realized I had fallen back into the cycle I had worked so hard to get out of just a few years prior. I knew then that I could not weigh myself anymore. I committed to myself that I would never again, out of my own free will, know the number on the scale.

If you have taken *The Love Your Body Class* from me or worked with me one on one, you have heard me say that the scale is the devil! I truly believe this.

Today, I am proud to say that I do not know the exact number of my weight. I do not want to know. I have no desire to know. It does not matter to me. I am happiest and the most free this way.

When I go to the doctor and they check me in, they always take my blood pressure, check my height, and put me on the scale.

I always tell the nurse, "I would like to stand backwards, please, so I do not see the number, and please do not record the number down on my sheet so that I can see it. Knowing the number makes me crazy."

A typical response I get is, "You don't look like you need to worry about your weight."

I respond with, "Thank you, but at one time I had an intense weight obsession, and not knowing my weight is one of the tools I use to stay free from it."

They never argue with me after that. I understand it may be an odd request, but I don't care! My mental freedom means more to me than what any nurse or any other person thinks for that matter.

So I challenge you to throw away your scale, your tape measure, and anything else you use to check your body. Make a commitment to never buy one again. Make a commitment to not weigh yourself ever again.

If you choose to continue to weigh yourself at the gym or the doctor or wherever else a scale can be found, pay attention to what you are like when you are not weighing yourself and when you are. Do you think differently? Do you behave differently? When are you really honest with yourself? When are you more at peace?

This is one of the most important tools I have in my toolbox and one of the most important tools that I can offer you! Weighing yourself does not create a friendly relationship with your body. When you weigh yourself, you are judging your body EVERY time, and whether you feel good or bad about the number you see, your body takes it as not being good enough... unless... unless it is a certain weight.

Would you tell your lover they are not worthy of your love unless they hit a certain number on the scale??? The answer is no. At least I hope you would never treat the person you love that way.

What would your relationship with your body be like if you did not weigh in?

How much more freedom would you experience if you did not weigh in?

How much easier would it be to listen to what your body needs when you are not worried about numbers on a scale?

What if throwing the scale out brought you freedom?

What if you actually lost weight after you threw your scale out?

What would it take for you to throw your scale out?

What would it take for you to commit to never knowing the number on the scale ever again?

Ever!

Chapter 27

Get Out of the Mirror

The mirror can be similar to the scale. It is often used as another way to measure yourself. Does this sound familiar? You take a look in the mirror first thing in the morning to see if you are alright, to see if you are presentable, to see if you are worthy, and to see if you are lovable. You analyze and scrutinize the lining of your silhouette to see whether your stomach is protruding or not. You eye the sides of your hips. Are they bulging more or less this morning? It's just another way to continue an unkind relationship with your body.

From my experience, the mirror was another thing I had to "throw out" so to speak. No, I didn't literally throw out the mirrors around my house, but I chose not to use them as a source for analyzing my body. It wasn't easy, as I had conditioned myself to look at my body in every mirror I came across. I never passed up the chance to look at my reflection in a window from the side view. If I was walking on the street, I would always look into the reflection of store windows to see how flat my stomach was. If I was out at a restaurant or a bar, and I was alone in the bathroom with no one looking, I always pulled up my shirt so that I could see what my stomach looked like in that moment. I was always checking to make sure it was flat, and if it wasn't, I would feel like a failure. If I was wearing a dress, I would pull it up, so that I could see how my panties lay on my hips and if they cut into my hips at all. This was craziness, but it was a habit I had created, constantly checking to see if I was okay.

For years, my friends and family would tell me that I was crazy. I remember my sister would say it jokingly, imitating the sound of a coo coo clock. She would put her hands on the sides of her face and turn her head from side to side while saying, "Coo coo, coo coo."

It was always funny, but I always thought she was just being nice or she was the one that was coo coo if she could not actually see that I was fat and that I was not perfect!

There is a condition called body dysmorphic disorder, where someone actually sees a distorted image of their body and they literally do not see their body accurately for what it is. I think there are extreme cases of this and, of course, there are very mild cases as well.

How many times have you looked back at pictures and thought you looked great, but then remember that at the time you had thought you were so fat? I'm not saying that's body dysmorphic disorder, I'm just saying that sometimes we have a skewed outlook on how we actually look.

Is it possible that you do not see your body shape accurately? I have had clients tell me that they think they look smaller in the mirror and then see themselves as much larger in pictures. When you are preoccupied with your weight, is it likely or unlikely that you are viewing yourself accurately and honestly?

Eventually, I resolved to use the mirror to put my makeup on, brush my teeth, brush my hair, to check that my shoes go with my outfit, and to check that I look polished as a whole before leaving the house. I began choosing not to use the mirror to see what my body looks like so that I could judge it.

Why do people judge their own bodies and say unkind words, but they don't say unkind things to the people they love and care about?

For example, you would probably never say to your best friend before she leaves the house, "Come here, and let me look at you. Oh my God! Your thighs look big in that outfit. You seriously need to stop eating when you say you are going to! Go change! There is no way I am going to be seen with you looking like that!"

What would this do to your relationship with your friend? It would likely drive a wedge between the two of you. She would be hurt and angry at you and she would not want to be kind back to you in any way. She probably wouldn't even want to speak with you or spend time with you. This is the same with your relationship with your body. If you wouldn't talk to your friend like that, why would you talk to yourself in that way?

Remember, when you are kind to your body, your body is kind to you. When you are loving to your body, your body is loving to you. When you honor your body, your body honors you.

I have found it is best for me to have a neutral attitude about my weight, one where I am not thinking about whether it is good or bad for any reason, just that it is. It just is my body. It just is my beautiful body that gifts me in this life with the ability to walk, run, breathe, smile, brush my teeth, drive a car, give kisses, hear music, smell the scent of a man, etc.

It is my beautiful body no matter what size it is, period.

Be aware of how you use the mirror or anything that you can see your reflection in. Are you analyzing your body? What are you saying to yourself as you are looking in the mirror? What messages are you telling yourself? Don't use the mirror to measure yourself. It will keep you in *The Abuse Your Body Cycle.*

I have found that any judgment in the mirror is not being kind to the body. If you are telling it how skinny it is and how happy you are about it, you are giving your body the message that it is loved if… it looks like this…

We need to love and appreciate our bodies, simply because they are our bodies, and also for the gifts they give us. Choose something kind to say to yourself when you look in the mirror to replace the old negative self-talk. I have always used, "I love my body, my body is beautiful."

Choose to tell yourself something you would like to believe.

Getting out of the mirror is not avoiding anything. It is removing yourself from a situation that is harmful to your spirit. Someone that is addicted to gambling and has decided to stop does not go to a casino, sit at a Blackjack table, but then choose to not play. Why would they do that? So, choose to use the mirror only when you need it and not to analyze or measure your body.

Chapter 28

Messages from the Media

I am appalled by all of the ads that are out there constantly bombarding people about how they are not good enough and encouraging them that if they just lost 5 pounds they would be happy. On top of that, I am horrified by the way the general public has bought this idea as truth and has helped to spread this idea.

I have noticed that many people post online about food, weight, and body image. I once saw a post that eluded to the idea that it takes a lot of strength to control what goes on one's plate throughout the day. Many people related to this post, encouraging this type of thinking, and sharing it with others.

Controlling anything is a lot of work and takes away one's freedom to choose. When you take away the freedom to choose from a human being, they automatically want to break free from that restriction. This is why controlling your food has great potential to eventually lead to breaking promises to yourself.

I wonder what would go on your plate if you asked your body what it wanted to eat and you listened to it, versus if you were telling it what it can eat and can't eat, and trying to control it. What do you think would happen? Let's pretend those two plates existed. What would be on those plates at the end of the day? I'm going to paint a scenario of one person's day that listens to their body and another scenario of someone who is constantly trying to control their weight.

A person that listens to their body would probably have a day like this: In the morning they would go into the kitchen, open the fridge and say, "Hmmm, body, what looks good to you? What would you like to eat today?"

And then their body would say, "An egg, toast, and an orange for breakfast sounds satisfying," and so they would eat the egg, toast, and orange, and then go on with their day.

Their stomach would feel good and they would have the energy they need to get themselves through the morning.

When it is time for lunch, they leave their desk and go get the salad with French bread that they had brought with them to work, and they ask, "Body, would you like to eat this salad and bread for lunch?"

The answer is yes.

By the way, if the answer was no, and they have time to get something else for lunch, then that is an option they could choose. If there is not enough time, then they can bless the food, pray over it, and ask for the food to become what their body needs for nourishment. (Refer to the chapter on *There is No Waste*.)

After lunch, they are re-energized for the afternoon's work and food is no longer on their mind while they are working.

For dinner, they are meeting a friend out. They look at the menu and they ask their body, "Body, what would you like to eat tonight for dinner?" and as they scan the menu, the teriyaki salmon with rice and green beans pops out to them, and their body says, "Yeah, that looks good."

So they order the salmon dish, and enjoy it completely, because that is what their body requires of them.

In contrast, the person that is controlling their body would probably start the day out with a preconceived notion of what they should or should not be having for breakfast in order to lose weight or not gain weight. A likely breakfast for this person might consist of an energy bar.

After they consume the energy bar, they think of what they can't eat all the way until lunch time. Although, they have already snuck a few chocolate pieces from the receptionist's desk, which they justify in their head doesn't count since it was just a few pieces and no one saw them eat them.

Then for lunch they have their veggies and fat-free ranch with a piece of string cheese wrapped inside a piece of lettuce and deli turkey. It isn't very satisfying to them, and they are still hungry when they finish their meal, but they believe that they must eat this way if they are going to lose weight or at the least not gain weight.

Then the afternoon rolls around and they are so hungry and light-headed from the lunch of deprivation, that they tell themselves they just need to have a little something, so they go to the vending machine with the intention of finding a healthy snack and they choose the trail mix, but after eating the trail mix, they decide it just wasn't satisfying. They are still hungry when they go back to their desk, and they can't stop thinking about how what they really wanted from the vending machine was the bag of potato chips in the first place. They justify in their head that it is only one bag of chips, telling themselves that if they don't eat it they won't be able to work because they still feel lightheaded and hungry, so they purchase the bag of potato chips and eat that too, feeling okay about their decision while they are eating it. Immediately after they finish the chips, they begin to feel guilty. They just blew their diet!!! The bag of chips totally ruined their diet! They decide that they will never do that again and that tonight for dinner they will have no carbs!!!

They go out to dinner with their friend with the full intention of ordering a salad with light dressing and no carbs to go along with it, but then they smell the aroma of all the hearty food being served to people at their tables and they think, and think, and they go back and forth in their head on whether or not they should order a side of fries with their salad because they know if they just have the salad with no carbs they will be hungry. Then they decide that tomorrow they will start their diet over and tonight they will have that grilled chicken sandwich with French fries (and a side of guilt). They eat all of it, even though it was too much food, and as they are finishing up their dinner conversation with their friend, they start thinking about how full they are, and how they can never stick to any diet, and how if they could just lose those last 10 pounds then they would have no problems at all. They start thinking about how they really blew it, but tomorrow they will start their diet all over and be good. Since they are starting their diet over tomorrow, they order the brownie sundae for dessert and have that too.

Does that sound familiar?

So, the person who was not preoccupied with their weight, and asked their body what it wanted to eat, ate:

An egg, toast, and an orange

French bread and a salad

Salmon, rice and green beans

The person who was pre-occupied with their weight, and made decisions based on what they should and shouldn't be eating, ate:

Energy bar

A few chocolate pieces

Veggies, cheese, turkey

Trail mix

Potato chips

Chicken sandwich and fries

Brownie sundae

Usually people who are dieting or pre-occupied with their weight, tend to eat more than those who are not pre-occupied with their weight and not dieting. People who ask their body what it would like, tend to eat less than people who are following their bought beliefs of what they should and shouldn't eat.

Another post I saw on the internet lately was a picture of a woman in stages of getting skinnier and it talked about following a program to lose bad weight. The post actually used the words "bad weight."

Bad weight? That's an interesting point of view. Do you see how this industry is brainwashing everyone to hate their bodies??? They are making tons of money off of you hating your body, dieting, losing weight, regaining it, paying to go on another one of their fad diets or take their pills; losing the weight and then regaining it. They are profiting from your self-hatred. It's incredible!

I can see this because I have been removed from it for a very long time and it now pisses me off! It pisses me off because I know way too many people who are not enjoying their lives because all they can think about is their weight. I understand this; I lived it for 20 years.

Then there are celebrities who have *lost the weight and kept it off.* What happens when you see an advertisement on the internet about a celebrity's weight loss and you click on that link? It takes you to a page where you can buy a product!!! Their purpose is to make money off of you.

Pay attention to the media and what you are being told, and what people are saying about themselves, including your friends on social media. Awareness changes everything. When you start to notice how you are being bombarded with messages from all around you, including many forms of media, you will begin to question if what you have believed about your body not being good enough is true or not.

What if what you believe about your body, didn't actually come from you?

What if the thought of you believing that your body is not good enough, came from somewhere else or someone else?

What if you stopped buying the idea that you are not perfect?

What if your body is perfect as it is right now?

What if what society says is a perfect body, is just a point of view that someone created and is selling to you so that they can make money off you and your misery?

What would it take for you to stop buying the point of view that you're not good enough and that your body is not perfect?

What would your life be like if you believed your body is perfect and beautiful as it is?

What would your life be like if you saw your body as the gift that it is?

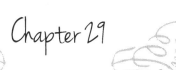

Chapter 29

Throw it Out-Your Magazines

Chances are, if you are obsessed with your weight, you also have a tendency to be drawn to magazines on fitness, or articles on how the next miracle diet will end your weight issue, where you are promised to lose 15 pounds in a week if you just eat soup or cut out carbs or add 2 miracle foods to your diet; or magazines that display article titles such as, "Tone up those abs in just 5 minutes a day."

I used to subscribe to a few of those magazines, but I stopped subscribing and reading them when I realized that they were contributing to my poor body image and weight obsession. I tried every diet they offered, and yes, if I stuck to the diet, I would lose some weight, but the moment I went and "failed" or "messed up" or "fell off the wagon," I would put it all back on or more because I felt like I had already lost.

I also stopped reading magazines that are full of skinny supermodels and actors and actresses. Why? Because I was always comparing myself to them. In my head, I thought that they were the ideal, that they were what I was supposed to be and look like, and no matter how hard I tried, I never got to look like them. I realized much later, that I don't have an airbrush like their editors do. Those pictures are not real. They are not real! They are touched up. All cellulite is touched up, and model's arms, legs, and stomachs are touched up and taken in.

I say no to reading magazines that have pictures of "perfect" bodies, and diets and workouts that promise I will be a perfect me if I just follow what they say.

I used to cut out pictures of models that had the type of body I wanted. I would put these images on my mirror so I would see them every morning when getting ready, to remind me that I needed to stick to my diet. Let's be honest, I didn't need a reminder, it was all I thought about anyway. I also thought it would have a subliminal effect on my mind to lose weight. On top of that, I would post those pictures on my fridge as a reminder that I wanted to be skinny, and so that I wouldn't eat too much, in an effort to remind me to make a "good" choice. All it actually did was remind me that I didn't look like them. I'd been trying for a long time to look like those supermodels and celebrities.

Anything that enables you or encourages you to compare yourself to another about how you look or the size of your body is not kind. It is only reinforcing your self-loathing and deepening the rift between you and your relationship with your body, so be kind to your body and don't compare it to someone who is airbrushed and modified in a magazine.

For me, giving up the magazines was much easier than giving up my scale, but I found it was another tool that helped me cure the obsession. Now, when I see that type of media, I laugh and think what a gimmick it is. They are just trying to make another buck off selling you their ideas, based on your insecurities, habits, and obsessions which likely began as a result of reading and buying into what they started telling you in the first place years ago.

If reading these types of magazines resulted in a happier you then I would say, by all means read them. But, do they contribute to your happiness? Do they contribute to the relationship you have with your body in a happy, healthy, and positive way? If following a "healthy" diet from a magazine leads to you "falling off the wagon" later and binging and purging or even just talking hatefully to yourself, would you consider that to be a positive contribution to your wellbeing?

I know it may be tough at first to say no to those magazines, they can be fun to read and have great articles, but if they are not contributing positively, think about how they are contributing to you.

Today I can say I have been magazine free for over a decade. I don't read those types of magazines anymore, and I don't miss them either. I guess it's kind of like sugar for me. I don't eat it anymore and I don't miss something that made me feel bad about myself.

If you are anything like me, you can't stand the thought of sitting through one more bullshit advertisement telling you how you can lose those 10 pounds of fat in the next 7 days! If you are anything like me, you are sick and tired of the bullshit! Dieting is NOT fun anymore and you don't believe a word that those people are trying to sell you anymore. If you are anything like me, you have had enough of trying to get *there*, and you have had enough of being brainwashed that you are only good enough if you look a certain way.

How are the things you are choosing to read contributing to your well-being?

Chapter 30

When You Start Changing Behaviors

When you start changing your behaviors and changing the way you choose to view food and weight, you may not always feel comfortable. For the first time, you may have to deal with situations where you usually would have run to food in order to cover up or stuff your emotions, or where you might have punished yourself with deprivation or purging, and this may feel uneasy to you. Instead of fighting feelings of uneasiness and trying to get rid of them, soak into them, go towards them. Remember, your body is letting you know something through a feeling, it is communicating with you, telling you that you are doing something different and it's not used to it, it's not comfortable with it, and it's a little scary.

And that's okay.

Acknowledge whatever it is that you are feeling. Perhaps it's, "Yes, I feel uneasy in my skin. It is scary for me to not use food, calorie counting, different forms of purging, etc."

A question you can ask is, "What can I do for me to be kind and loving to me right now?"

A question that I have also used when I don't feel comfortable is, "What part of me is coming up that I do not know?"

Why this question? Because if I have used food, deprivation, or any substance for that matter to cover my feelings, then there are parts of me that I have buried or covered for so long that I do not know.

Then when you have the energy of what came up after you asked that question, say, "You are safe here, it's safe for you to be here."

It's not easy feeling uncomfortable when you are changing the way you choose, but when you are too full physically or feeling guilty or hating your body, that is not exactly a feeling of comfort either, is it? The fact of the matter is that you will not feel comfortable 24 hours a day in life, period, but when you don't feel comfortable, try to just be with that feeling and acknowledge it. It will pass. It's there to teach you something or to show you something about your life. Be kind to yourself.

As you practice being with your feelings instead of fighting them, this will become a natural reaction to unease, and this will contribute to breaking *The Abuse Your Body Cycle*.

Chapter 31

Punishments and Rewards

Food is meant to be eaten so that we can sustain our life and have the energy we need to continue living. Of course, you can enjoy the food you eat. Food has different tastes and food can be pleasurable. But when you eat to reward yourself, you are using food for something other than its main purpose.

For someone who does not have a weight obsession, they may be able to reward themselves here and there with something, but for someone who has a weight obsession, this can contribute to *The Abuse Your Body Cycle* and here's why.

Someone who has a weight obsession and is constantly on a diet or watching their weight will reward themselves with food and also punish themselves with food. Someone who eats "normally" may reward themselves with food, but they don't punish themselves with food, and this is the key difference. Once they have "rewarded" themselves that is the end of the story. They will not think about what they ate after they have eaten it. They won't count calories. They won't worry whether what they ate will put on weight or not. The meal is over once they have stopped eating it. They also do not reward themselves with something they think is bad, whereas someone who has an issue with food and weight will.

For example, let's say the person without the weight obsession gets a job promotion. They may call their friend and say, "Guess what, I got the promotion at work today, let's go out and celebrate at a nice restaurant tonight."

This person is celebrating their achievement of getting promoted with the reward of being with their friend and going out to a nice restaurant. They are not thinking about what they are going to choose to eat that they normally try to stay away from because it is "bad" for them. They won't overindulge in food that they wouldn't normally choose to eat anyway, because they don't have the point of view that there is food that makes them fat and food that doesn't.

When the evening comes and they go to dinner, they order as they normally do, they eat as they normally would, maybe they order an entrée that costs more than they would normally spend and maybe they order a dessert. They are satisfied when they leave the table and their life goes on. There is no more thought about what they ate. The reward is the going out to dinner with a friend.

Now, let's look at an example from the person who has the weight obsession. This person has been on a diet for a few weeks and has been really good at sticking with it and following all of the rules of the diet. They have lost a few pounds and they are happy to be in control of their weight once again. This person gets the promotion at work and thinks to themselves that they want to celebrate at a nice restaurant. They call their friend, "Guess what, I got the promotion at work today, let's go out and celebrate at a nice restaurant tonight."

At the restaurant, this person thinks how hard they have worked for this promotion and how they have been so "good" on this diet, that just for tonight they can splurge and have it all. They order the foods that are on their "naughty" list. They leave the table feeling a little too full and with that old familiar feeling of guilt lingering in their mind. They blew their diet! That night as they are lying in bed, all they can think about is how they hope that dinner does not put on a couple of pounds after all of the hard work and deprivation that they have put themselves through.

The next morning, they wake up and they still feel guilty. They are extra determined today to cut their calories from this diet in half to make up for last night's splurge and celebration. Another way of putting this is that now they will punish themselves after the reward. This person will make one of two choices after last night's reward. They will continue on their diet while cutting back on food the following day or they will feel hopeless that they messed up, fall off their diet, and continue to make choices that make them feel guilty until they can pull it together again to go on another diet. The reward was the splurge. The punishment is the cut in calories the next day, the mind beating, or falling off the diet, and continuing to feel guilty and hopeless because they just can't seem to get it right.

Do you see the difference between the two types of thinking? People who are weight obsessed will most likely punish themselves after they reward themselves. It's part of *The Abuse Your Body Cycle*. They are not even aware of what they are doing.

If you have a celebration in your life, rejoice in that celebration with your heart, with gratitude, or in a way that is serving to your spirit and your body. Get a massage, go for a walk, call and share your news with those you love. I'm not saying don't go out to dinner, but if you do, don't reward yourself with food. Why on this day would your wonderful body deserve to eat something different than any other day? For people who are obsessed with their weight, rewards often come with punishment.

Another way I see people reward themselves with food is when they are doing well on a diet and have lost weight. They will "cheat" or reward themselves with a particular food that they believe is bad: fries, cake, pizza, whatever it is. But that reward will most likely lead to guilt and punishment.

Be aware of the next time you think about rewarding yourself with food, and if you choose to reward yourself with food, be aware of what happens afterwards. I highly recommend not using food as a reward.

Another way I have seen people reward themselves is on vacation. Why would you choose to eat any differently on vacation than you would any other day? One of my newer clients recently sent me an email after she had been on a two week vacation and she said, "Since I ate normally on my vacation, I don't need to go on a diet now that I am back. I just used the tools. This is my first vacation where I didn't put on any weight."

She did not need to punish herself because she did not reward herself for being on vacation. She just used her tools every day, and asked her body how she would feel after she ate something. She felt good in her body and knew that she did not gain any weight on vacation from over-indulging just because she was on vacation.

If you are asking your body what it wants to eat, then it shouldn't need to be rewarded, because every meal and every choice is a happy one for the body.

What are some ways that are non-food related that you would like to reward yourself in the future when the time comes?

Chapter 32

Forgiveness and Grace

In a relationship between two people, forgiveness and grace help to heal wounds, misunderstandings, and unkind actions or words.

What about forgiving yourself for the ways that you have treated your body? What about giving yourself grace for not doing everything perfectly? If you tell your body that you are sorry, will your body forgive you? Absolutely! Over time, it will begin to trust you and your choices because you are communicating with it in a loving way. How can you be sure that your body has forgiven you? Because eventually your body begins to heal itself from the past harm that you did to it. Whatever it was that you did to hurt your body, your body will begin healing. Your body is miraculous like that. Your body will forgive you. Isn't that incredible how generous, kind, and loving your body is to you? Your body will repair and heal past hurts you have done to it. Your body loves you!

I abused my body for many years. I would overeat, I would throw up my food, I would take laxatives, I would work out on a hurt knee, I would starve, and I told it so many unkind words. I had to tell my body, "I am so sorry that I abused you in this way. I choose not to throw up my food anymore. If I choose to put something in my mouth, then I am going to choose to keep it down and deal with the consequences of feeling too full or believing that it is going to put on weight."

I had to stick with that commitment after my apology in order to build trust with my body, and I did keep that commitment. It also helped me to be more mindful of my choices, because I knew that purging was no longer an option for me.

My throat that used to be sore returned to normal. The indigestion that I had, vanished. The discomfort and pain in my knee went away. The mind chatter left. My body repaired the damage I had caused. It forgave me. Lucky me! What a gift my body is!

Forgiveness is probably something that everyone can work on a little more in their life. Forgiving others and forgiving oneself. In general we are the most unkind to ourselves. We will be harder on ourselves than we will be on any other person. We will put ourselves down for multiple reasons and causes. Often, we do it throughout the day and we are not even aware of how we are talking to ourselves, and not just about our weight, but about our self-worth on so many levels.

For example, I tend to have many new ideas for creating new businesses. I will get really excited, and then I start to hear in my head, *Do you really think that you can do that?*

Or, if I attend a workshop or seminar I may think, *She is a way better public speaker than you are!*

I have had to tell myself, *Stop! You don't even teach the same thing! People need to hear what you are sharing with them. It's not about you, it's about the message,* and then I'll apologize to myself for being unkind.

How often are we hard on ourselves for the decisions that we have made?

When we speak unkindly to ourselves like that, what do you think that does to our body?

What we think has a direct effect on our body.

Have you ever thought like this after you ate?

I can't believe I just ate that large French fry. What was I thinking? Oh, that's right, I wasn't. Once again, if I see it, I eat it.

What kind of message is this? This message reinforces that if you see something, you eat it; a hopeless situation that you have no choice in. If you choose to alter your response, then what you do will also change. Instead try:

I just ate a large fry mindlessly. Body, I am so sorry that I did not check in with you. I will remember that I don't like the way I feel when

I do not think before I eat, and I will remind myself to check in with you prior to eating next time.

This message allows change to occur. You have brought awareness to the forefront of your mind to take care of your body; consider it and honor it.

You have two choices, you can be hard and unkind to yourself, or you can give yourself grace and forgiveness. You are not perfect, no one is, but you are perfect just as you are. You are not alone in not being perfect, but you are surrounded by people who are perfect just as they are.

As you start giving out forgiveness and grace to yourself, start giving it to others too. You will find that people are attracted to your love and generosity of grace. The more you are kind and loving to yourself, the more others will want to be in your presence.

Chapter 33

There is No Perfect Relationship

There is no perfect relationship; not with your wife, not with your husband, not with your best friend, not with your sister, not with your brother, not with yourself, and not with your body. However, there are good relationships and there are healthy relationships. Relationships don't stay the same either. They change and grow over time. Life events affect the stability of relationships, and life events can make relationships stronger or make them weaker. Sometimes a life event occurs and we feel distant from our partner, or we feel unloved, neglected or forgotten. We begin to distance ourselves from our partner, but that doesn't mean that we love them less or that there isn't hope. How we treat those we love during these times makes all the difference in our ability to heal our relationship.

This too can happen with our relationship with our body. Things can be going great. We can feel really solid in our relationship with our body and be very confident. We may even be so confident that we think we are completely past it and find ourselves feeling secure when looking back on how we used to overeat, or used to starve, or used to binge and purge, or used to obsess over weight, but then one day maybe months or years later, we notice we are looking in the mirror again judging our body, or looking at a package to count the calories, or counting the hours until our next meal.

It may start out slowly. You might say to yourself, "Just this one time I will look in the mirror at my body."

"Just this one time, I will look at how many calories are in that tortilla."

"Just this one time, I will count how many hours until my next meal."

Then the next thing you notice, you seem to be back into your old thought patterns and fighting your old behaviors. The good news is, you are now aware of these patterns and have the tools to not let yourself go back into the cycle of abuse. You have the tools, you know how to talk to yourself, you know how to choose, and you know how to go back to basics.

It is important to ask yourself, "What happened?"

"Did something occur to affect my relationship with my body?"

"Why did I start going into old thought patterns?"

"Why was I attracted to those old ways of thinking and doing?"

Most likely something happened in your life that affected your relationship with your body. Something changed to disrupt the flow that you were in. Something occurred for you in your life that made you become careless or disconnected in your relationship with your body, without you even being aware of it at the time. There is nothing "wrong" with this. Just as when you have a relationship or friendship with someone, there can be misunderstandings and life events that affect those relationships. If you have the tools and the desire to heal your relationships, you usually find a way.

Some of the life events that can affect your relationship with your body are: getting a new job, moving your residence, someone close to you dies, you give up an addiction, or you go on a vacation.

There are a number of things that can affect your relationship with your body and make you feel disconnected or out of sorts. The good news is that you recognize it and it's important that you do something with what you recognize. Knowledge is only power if you take action.

If and when this happens, ask your body, "What can I do to honor you?"

Take more care with your body. Be extra appreciative towards your body. Acknowledge and thank it for all of the gifts it gives you.

When you recognize that something has changed in your relationship with your body or you are going back to old patterns, go back to basics.

Chapter 34

Back to Basics

When I find that I am disconnected in my relationship to my body, I remind myself to go back to the basics. What are the basics? For me the basics are: not judging my body in the mirror, not counting calories, not counting time from my last meal until my next meal, definitely not weighing myself, choosing what to eat by asking how I will feel after I eat it, and being very present with what I choose to eat. It's slowing down and acknowledging that I need to pay more attention to this relationship in my life, lest it slip away and one day I don't recognize it anymore.

It's like going back to the beginning of a relationship when the man first starts courting the woman and both man and woman are very aware of how they are taking care of each other. There is no routine established yet in the relationship. By going back to basics, you are extra aware of how you are treating your relationship with your body. You give it extra time and extra care. Please understand that I believe relationships should always be cared for and nurtured, but it is also normal to be in a healthy relationship that has found its comfort and its routine in a healthy flow. Just as we have seasons of weather, we have seasons in relationships.

The times I have found that I have needed to go back to the basics were because I had stopped trusting my body for some reason or another. Usually, I didn't know why I had stopped trusting, but when I would look back on that time in my life later, I was able to pinpoint that I had a big change occur in my life, and that big change resulted in a death of a part of myself and a rebirth of another part of myself.

For example, when I had truly quit smoking, there were parts of me that I did not recognize as me. These parts of me showed up as anxiety, and I didn't know what to do with myself when I felt this anxiety, and sometimes I felt like eating. Thank God I had these tools because I was able to recognize that I didn't actually want to eat but that I was feeling uncomfortable in my skin because something that was a part of me was gone and I was grieving the loss of what this substance once meant to me.

Every time I felt anxiety or uneasiness, I would ask, "What part of me is coming up right now that I do not know?" and I would say, "You are welcome, you are safe here, and I'm sorry I suppressed you."

I spoke to myself this way because I had used smoking to suppress my feelings without even realizing it. I smoked when I was happy, angry, celebrating something, when I was nervous or just because, so I covered a lot of feelings and a lot of myself that I didn't even know I was covering. People do that with food too. Often they don't even know why they are opening the refrigerator door or going to purchase a snack from the vending machine at work and they just mindlessly eat.

Next time you find yourself mindlessly grabbing something to put in your mouth, ask, "Body, are you really hungry?"

Your body will let you know and it will bring your awareness to your stomach. When I use this tool, I find that 9/10 times I am not hungry, rather I am avoiding a situation or covering up a feeling that I was not even aware that I was feeling or avoiding. If your body says yes it is hungry, then great, ask your body what it would like to eat, (not your mind, your body), and enjoy it, sit down, be present with your food and delight in each bite. If your body tells you it is not hungry, you can ask, "Body, what is it that you want me to know right now?" or "What am I feeling or experiencing right now?"

You do not need to try and figure out all of the answers to these questions, you just need to ask, and your body and spirit together will let you know at the right time and in the right way, but these questions will stop you from mindlessly eating by bringing awareness to the situation.

You can ask your body any question that you feel is fit. Those are just some questions I ask my body. You are in a relationship with your body, so communicate in a way that feels good to you, and in a way that you are honoring your body. There is no right or wrong or one way to communicate, just go with what feels right. We are incredibly intuitive and gifted human beings, ALL of us.

When you are in doubt of what to do for your body relationship and you are feeling disconnected, go back to the basics.

- Choose not to judge your body in the mirror
- Choose not to count calories
- Choose not to count time
- Choose not to weigh yourself
- Ask your body what it would like to eat
- Be present with your food

Chapter 35

Being Skinny Doesn't Make You Happy

Being skinny doesn't make you happy. Feeling good about you makes you happy. I have heard from clients that when they had lost weight in the past, they were still unsatisfied and the goal became to lose more. One beautiful girl, during *The Love Your Body Class,* explained that she had lost 83 pounds in her journey and still was not happy; she still wanted to lose more.

You may be familiar with the scenario of, "If I could just lose 20 pounds, I'd be happy," or "If I could just lose 5 pounds, I'd be happy," and then when you get there, you're still not happy with your weight or how your body looks.

That is because losing weight goes deeper than just the weight loss. It may be a way to focus your energy on something else other than your life, or a way to stay disconnected from your body, or you have bought into the messages that are all around us from our society that you are not good enough if you are not emaciated, rich, young, and wrinkle-free. Being skinny doesn't make you happy, because the core issue is not the weight; the core issue is your belief system around the weight and your body.

Of course, people eat for emotional reasons, just as they smoke, drink, shop, gamble, and do drugs. I'm absolutely certain that therapy serves a purpose in this regard, but I also believe that when you build a relationship with your body and you begin to respect it, you no longer want to harm it, and you find other approaches to calm the chatter in your head, such as breathing techniques, moving your body, writing, speaking to your body, going towards what you feel instead of fighting it, and allowing the energy within you to be what it is.

When you have envy for another person that you think is thinner than you, has a better butt than you, or tighter arms, or just has a better body than you in general, you have no idea what that person's story is. You don't know what they have been through in their life. You don't know if they had bypass surgery in the past or liposuction or are currently in a state of starvation. When you find yourself judging someone else, wishing you have what they have, send that person love and light and bless them.

Happiness comes from being able to be you in the body that you currently have. You will find that you are able to be comfortable in the body that you have, when you build a healthy relationship with your body. It will feel good to be in your body, and it will feel good to feel your body.

I have clients that do not have the body shape that the media sells us to have, and they are very happy to be in their body. They love their bodies for everything that their bodies give them and they have let go of the expectations that the media and our society say we must be. They have taken the point of view that, *If you don't like me the way I am, I don't really care. Your judgments have nothing to do with my happiness and how I feel in my body.*

Have you ever been skinny before? Have you ever reached your "goal" weight?

You can feel fat at 95 pounds, 120 pounds, 150 pounds, 190 pounds, 250 pounds. You could have been 250 pounds and now you are 160 pounds, and you still feel fat. Once again, that is because it is not the number or the size that you are that makes you happy. It is what you believe and have bought into about what makes you a worthy and good person that makes you happy.

One afternoon in San Diego, I was walking to the beach and this hard-bodied guy approached me. He was trying to get my attention to start a conversation with me, so I engaged him just enough as he walked with me to see if I wanted to continue the conversation or not. His name was Steven.

When I had chosen my place on the sand and laid my towel out, he sat down next to me on the sand. As we continued to talk, I began to realize that all this guy cared about was his looks. He kept referring to how ripped and tight he was. When he asked me what I did, I didn't think it would resonate with him.

I said, "I work with people who are frustrated with their body and their weight and I teach them how to stop dieting and overeating and return to a normal and healthy lifestyle. I teach them how to love their body."

He winced. I mean he literally winced and then questioned, "You mean no matter what it looks like?"

I nodded my head.

He then said, "I don't agree with that at all. I work out every single day to look like this."

I just looked at him, smiled, and shrugged my shoulders, as if to say, "Okay, you don't have to."

There was a moment of silence, as I did not feel like engaging him in any kind of argument or winning him over to what I believe, because I have found people understand things when they are ready and if it's for them. My truth is not everyone's truth.

What happened next was interesting!

He said, "You know, I have a perfect body, but it doesn't do anything for me. I mean, yeah, I have strength when I surf. I can eat a lot of food. But having this perfect body doesn't really do anything for me. It doesn't even get me girls!"

I just watched him as he thought about what this perfect body he worked on every single day was doing for him. His brain was spinning as he was analyzing what this perfect hard body was getting him. He never mentioned what his body does for him on a daily basis. He only saw his perfect body as something that he is supposed to have and he brought up the belief that having a perfect body is supposed to get him chicks, but it actually didn't. Of course not, because, in the end, we're attracted to kindness, love, and a genuine spirit. Other than being strong for surfing, he didn't make any connection to health with his body.

He then went on for what felt like forever, but was probably only two minutes, about how he will never get down to 0% body fat no matter how hard he tries. In my head, I was like, *Who cares!!! What's the point?*

BORING! I was ready for him to leave my space and so I asked the universe, *What would it take for this guy to get up and go?*

I told him I had some work to do. He said goodbye and left me to my spot on the beach.

I share this story because this man made a really valid point, even having a "perfect" body according to what the media says is perfect, doesn't actually get you what you think it will. I understand the belief that, *When I have a perfect body I will attract more men,* or, *My husband will love me more,* or, *I will finally be happy.*

I understand because I have lived it, and I've seen it in so many people. What I also know is that I have been loved at all of my different weight levels and I have also been unloved at all of my different weight levels throughout my life. Just as I have been happy and unhappy at different weight levels. Weight is not the determinant of being liked and loved. Your heart is.

I had to ask, "What was the purpose of that guy coming into my world?"

My heart softened towards him as I remembered that he too is just a product of our world. I remembered that at one time, many, many years ago, I also thought I was great because of my body. I thought about the pressure he must put on himself to continue to look like he thinks he should because he's supposed to. I think that Steven and I both received a gift that day. He got to begin looking at why he does what he does and how his body serves him, and I got to have compassion for someone who is just doing what he believes he should do.

What is your perception about your body and how it correlates to your happiness?

Chapter 36

Your Weight is Going to Fluctuate-It's a Fact

One of the things that I had to accept was that my weight was going to fluctuate naturally. It had been my whole life, and no matter how much I tried to control it, I could never stop it completely.

There are those things that happen naturally, such as when a woman gets her period. It's almost inevitable she will be bloated and put on a few pounds. When a person travels in an airplane, they tend to retain water. Constipation can make one feel bloated. There are other life circumstances as well that can happen, like grieving and then losing your appetite. Those are all normal situations in which weight may fluctuate within a healthy range.

Since letting go, I have found that my weight definitely fluctuates. I don't know the numbers since I don't weigh myself, but I know because I will hear from people, "You look so skinny," or "Did you lose weight?"

My main response to people now when they comment on me looking thin is, "Oh that's interesting."

Years ago, I would have been so happy to hear that and I would have responded with, "Thank you."

But is it really a complement or is it a judgment on my body that someone else is making? I'm just throwing this question out there as something to ponder.

It was bizarre to me how a couple of months after my dad died, people were commenting on how skinny I was and asking me how I lost weight. My response was, "My dad died, I've been really depressed and I lost my appetite."

Remember when I wrote earlier in the book that you never know someone's story?

For me, my weight fluctuating is a result of me continuing on with my life and not worrying about it. I choose not to worry about it. I don't have the energy to beat myself up anymore.

In 2012, I spent a summer in Rome, Italy. While I was conscious of asking my body what it wanted to eat, I found I was eating a lot of pizza and a lot of pasta, plus I ate every meal out at a restaurant, except for breakfast. I had met an amazing man who took me out every other night to incredible dinners and the other nights I dined on my own or with friends I had made. Towards the end of my time there, I reached a point where I was like, "No more pizza and pasta!"

My body was tired of it. My body was now craving salads, big green salads with olives, tomatoes, mozzarella, and olive oil.

Towards the end of my time there, my clothes were a little snug on me. I told myself that it was okay. I had enjoyed my time in Italy, and would not hate myself for it. I told myself it was okay because I ate what I wanted, when my body wanted it. Was I perfect about asking my body what it wanted to eat all of the time? No, sometimes I forgot. And that's okay.

It was incredibly freeing to know that I chose what I ate without beating myself up. I also still loved and appreciated my body for all that it did for me. How could I not? That was the summer I had an experience that completely confirmed my appreciation for my body. That was the summer I was in the motorcycle accident, that I had mentioned earlier. While it was a minor accident, it awoke me to a whole other level of loving and appreciating my body.

My weight changes and I'm okay with that. It just is what it is, and I'm grateful my spirit has a healthy home.

Chapter 37

There is No There

At some point during my journey with weight obsession, I realized that I was never going to get *there* and stay *there*. I realized that I had always lost the weight only to see it return, and then I would lose it again, gain it back, lose it again and gain it back. I began to think that maybe I would be okay without all of the yo-yo dieting. I began to think that maybe my body would not be out of control, but would find its set point or a place that it liked to be. I also noticed that in the past when I had been really frustrated with dieting, and I wasn't on a diet, my body weight always seemed to go to a certain point, it seemed there was a place it liked to be at. I noticed that when I wasn't controlling my weight, I wasn't gaining weight as I had feared.

However, my natural set point is not super skinny or model skinny like I was trying to be all of those years when I was starving, binging and purging, and dieting. The natural set point of where my body likes to be is what I consider normal. It's my normal, and it's my perfect, and I like my body as it is now.

When you are constantly dieting and trying to control your weight, you are trying to get *somewhere*. You are trying to get *there*, but that *there* is only as good as your present moment. You cannot predict your future or your circumstances. When you are kind to your body and accept it as it is, in this moment, because this moment is your real *there*, you free yourself. It is in this space of now that you can finally start living and being. Trying to get *there* is a waste of energy.

A friend of mine recently went on a weight loss challenge. She worked out very hard and ate small portions, very small portions. She posted on Facebook that she will never again eat unhealthily and she will always be committed to exercise. I believe her intentions are good and she worked hard to get *there*, but her *there* is only as good as today. Nothing stays the same and everything is constantly changing and evolving.

I know people do this with happiness as well. They think when the anxiety they feel goes away, they will be happy. When they have a relationship, they will be happy. When they change jobs, they will be happy. When they get a new car, they will be happy. When they get a raise at work, they will be happy. Then they do get those things they wished for and they are still not content or satisfied or happy. If they are happy, it is for a short period of time and then they focus on the next thing that they think will make them happy. That is because satisfaction does not come from our future, it comes from the present moment and appreciating what we have right now, no matter what that looks like.

Naturally, we were born to strive for greatness and for more. It is good to make wise and thoughtful choices today that affect your future, but it is just as important to appreciate where you are now and what you have now. Your now is your *there*.

What would your life be like if you gave up getting your body *there*, which doesn't exist anyway, and if you accepted your body as it is here, because here was your *there* at some point in the past?

Gratitude is a quick and easy way to bring yourself from the *there* to your present moment. Whenever you catch yourself thinking about how great your life will be when you drop 10 pounds, or get a promotion at work, or take a vacation, start thanking God and the Universe for everything you can possibly think of that you have now.

"Thank you God that I can move my body."
"Thank you God for this water I drink."
"Thank you God for the support I have in my life."

"Thank you Universe for the air I breathe."

"Thank you Universe for my car that takes me places."
"Thank you Universe for the money in my wallet."

Gratitude wakes you up to the life you are living now. When you are grateful and express your gratitude, you will notice the Universe blessing you with gifts that you never even expected. Gratitude is really like a magic wand.

What would your life be like if you gave up getting your body there?

What would your life be like if you were grateful for what you have now and here?

How much more of your own life would you get to experience if you were functioning from here and not there?

What can you be thankful for in your life today, in this present moment?

Chapter 38

We Have to Be the Change

As we all know and are very aware of, we live in a world that bombards us with messages and judgments that we are not good enough. We have to be the change together. Each one of us, sharing with others how to treat ourselves with kindness and love, and how to treat others with the same. Setting an example is the best place to start and then spreading the word.

Compliment people for who they are, not for how skinny they look or how you have noticed they have lost weight. Compliment people for the gifts they bring into the world and the gifts they bring into your life. Compliment them for the gift they are.

In the end, we all just want to be loved. This is what people are striving for when they are trying so hard to look a certain way. They may have tons of things to show off, but it's not enough, because love doesn't come from what we look like or our material possessions. Love comes from within us.

I see the world changing. I see consciousness happening. I see more and more people who are aware of how their thoughts affect them and those around them. I see more and more people choosing love. I believe that every day our world gets healthier as each one of us does our part to give love to ourselves and love to others.

When I taught elementary school, I used to always tell my second and third graders, "Kindness is one of the greatest gifts we can give to another human being."

And guess what? It doesn't even cost you a dollar. It's free.

I will close with stating my vision once more:

My vision is that men and women, adults and children, throughout the world, will know their worth and beauty because of who they are and who they be; an incredible, beautiful, and lovable spirit; and that they love, nurture, and honor their earthly home, their gift, their BODY.

Will you join me and so many others in creating this movement by being the movement?

I always ask, "What would your life be like if you loved your body?"

Now, I'm also asking, "What would our world be like if men and women, adults and children, loved their bodies?"

It's just a choice.

With love and the deepest of gratitude,

Lemuela Christina

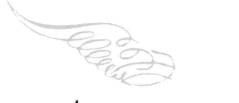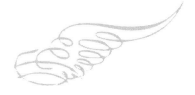

An invitation for you!

I have created a virtual book club for you, my reader, so that you can continue to use the tools in this book and grow your relationship with your body.

It's my gift to you (and free)!

I look forward to personally connecting with you through tele-calls, videos, articles, and more on how you can continue to build a healthy and happy relationship with your body.

You can sign up at www.lemuelachristina.com.

Visit www.lemuelachristina.com to learn more about the following classes and services.

The Lose the Guilt and Lose the Weight Class
The Love Your Body Breakthrough Session
The Love Your Body Private Session Retreat
The Love Your Body Class
The Love Your Body Group Coaching

If you would like me to speak at your organization, please contact me through email at lc@lemuelachristina.com.

About the Author

Lemuela Christina Duskis was born in Pasadena, California, and has spent most of her life living between Colorado and California. She has a wild passion for travel and has been to over 65 countries in her lifetime. Lemuela moved to Rome in 2013 to study the Italian language full-time, and it was there that the "Love Your Body" concept ripened. She taught her first class in her living room in Rome, where she felt compelled to share the tools she used to free herself from her weight obsession. Currently, her classes are taught in Colorado, California, and online.

Lemuela's gift for teaching others comes from her natural love of teaching and her training as an educator. She graduated with a Bachelor's of Science in Psychology in 2000 from Colorado State University in Fort Collins, Colorado, and received a Master's Degree in Cross Cultural Education in 2005 from National University in San Diego, California.

Lemuela believes that education is a major contributor to a happy and healthy life. This is why her mission is to educate people on how to love their body, through her classes, private sessions, and group coaching.

At present, Lemuela lives in San Diego, California.

Proof

Made in the USA
Charleston, SC
14 June 2016